Mometrix
TEST PREPARATION

Ophthalmology
Exam Secrets
Study Guide
Part 2 of 2

DEAR FUTURE EXAM SUCCESS STORY

First of all, **THANK YOU** for purchasing Mometrix study materials!

Second, congratulations! You are one of the few determined test-takers who are committed to doing whatever it takes to excel on your exam. **You have come to the right place.** We developed these study materials with one goal in mind: to deliver you the information you need in a format that's concise and easy to use.

In addition to optimizing your guide for the content of the test, we've outlined our recommended steps for breaking down the preparation process into small, attainable goals so you can make sure you stay on track.

We've also analyzed the entire test-taking process, identifying the most common pitfalls and showing how you can overcome them and be ready for any curveball the test throws you.

Standardized testing is one of the biggest obstacles on your road to success, which only increases the importance of doing well in the high-pressure, high-stakes environment of test day. Your results on this test could have a significant impact on your future, and this guide provides the information and practical advice to help you achieve your full potential on test day.

Your success is our success

We would love to hear from you! If you would like to share the story of your exam success or if you have any questions or comments in regard to our products, please contact us at **800-673-8175** or **support@mometrix.com**.

Thanks again for your business and we wish you continued success!

Sincerely,
The Mometrix Test Preparation Team

Need more help? Check out our flashcards at:
http://MometrixFlashcards.com/Ophthalmology

Written and edited by the Mometrix Exam Secrets Test Prep Team
Printed in the United States of America

TABLE OF CONTENTS

Neuro-Ophthalmology

First Questions to Ask

Begin with a sequential order of the patient's history. Start by asking the patient when his eyes last felt as though they were fine. Be vigilant in finding out exactly when the problem began. You may ask questions such as:

- At what point did the problem begin?
- Prior to that point, did you have eyes that were fine?
- Have you previously had a normal ocular check-up before the problem started? This may even have been for a driving examination or military assessment.
- Is there anything else?

Go on to take the person's interim history. Ask questions such as:

- What occurred next? Take an account of the problem.
- Have you gotten worse, better, or has the problem remained the same? Take an account of all information. Find out if the problem is the same, worsening with time, acute, partly acute, or ongoing.

Drugs and Societal Information

Regarding drugs – Find out what existing and prior medications the patient has. Get the amount of these drugs as well. Be sure to include non-prescription medications, herbal or unconventional medications, medications for birth control, aspirin, vitamins, or drops for the eyes.

Regarding societal information – Find out about the person's job, nutrition, use of tobacco or alcohol, vacation, animals, sexual record, and allergic reactions.

Once this information is taken, go back to reassess the history, making sure you are clear about the way the problem has gone for the patient and what his main complaint actually is. Go over the problem one more time, and then ask relevant questions regarding the complaints. Discover the main problems and warning signals.

One and a half syndrome – Both an abrasion of PPRF or sixth-nerve nucleus (resulting in one side having horizontal gaze palsy) and INO abrasion; both are located on the same side. This is caused by lack of blood flow to the brainstem, MS, tumor, bleeding in pons, or injury.

Afferent System Information

Get details regarding the following:

- When the symptoms begin each time
- Series of developments (quick beginning or a steady worsening)
- Length of time of the problem
- Rigorousness of lessened visual acuity, including asking questions such as:
  - Are you able to see someone's face?
  - Are you able to read?
- When the lessened visual acuity happened
- Worse on one side or the other
- Single eye / two eyes

- Steady worsening
- Problem in the field of vision vs. lessened visual acuity
- Linked hurting, which may be when the person moves the eyes, or may be in the form of pain in the head, queasiness, or aura
- Linked problem with motor or sensory abilities
- Linked scintillations or occurrences with the sense of sight

Torsional nystagmus – Goes in a roundabout motion; could also be up-and-down or side-to-side.

Afferent Localization and Hurting

Regarding afferent localization – Find out where the abrasion is located. Determine double vision in one or both eyes (vertical or horizontal). Determine if the problem is worse in fields of gaze so that the eyes are misaligned in every direction. Determine if the patient's problem deteriorates as the day goes by or not.

Regarding hurting – Determine the extent of the pain, the location of it, and the time that it happens. Find out if there is something that alleviates the problem but does not cure it. Find out what brings the hurting. Get accounts of other indications which are linked to this pain.

Convergence-retraction nystagmus – Occurring at the same time, but not in sync; generally back and forth, divided, yet joining together of cocontraction saccades. The cause will be different for different stages in the lifespan, as follows: infants - infant aqueductal stenosis; a ten year old - pinealoma; twenty-year - injury; thirty-year old - brainstem AVM; 40 year old - MS; fifty-year old - basilar artery stroke.

Neuroophthalmology Eye Examination

Point one – Visual acuity

- Put a patch on the unaffected eye to make sure the exam is correct. This is particularly important when examining a child's eye.
- Most excellent neutralization of vision problems utilizing Snellen
- Cycloplegic assessment with a retinoscope
- Overrefract when there are high powers to contend with
- Pinhole sight could be better than corrected visual acuity
- Assess sight for both near and far
- The visual acuity for both near and far ought to be equal
- Make a record of near vision
- Make a record of how fast the eye responds
- When vision is not good, assess how the eye sees light, movement, and directions
- If the patient is too young to talk or cannot talk, use optokinetic nystagmus (OKN) drum to evaluate

Point two – Balance of afferent system from one eye to the other:

- Balance of how quickly the response is
- Red desaturation; compare one eye to the other
- Brightness; look at each eye individually and then compare
- Evaluation of how the eye sees color; utilize Hardy-Rand-Rittler or Ishihara color plates

Point three – The pupil:

- Numerous assessments of the pupil
- Use equivalent light stimulation for both the right and left eyes
- Evaluate the dimensions, shape, light, and near reactions
- Utilize a strong light supply from underneath
- Check for afferent pupillary defect
- Evaluate the direct reaction for the right and left eye
- Move a flashlight from one eye to the other
- Look at ipsilateral dilation of the pupil after using the flashlight

Point four – External assessment:

- Take exophthalmos measurements
- Lid situation and how it is working
- Space between the margins of the lids
- Levator utility
- Margin-reflex distance
- Lid crease
- Low energy
- Lid retraction or lag
- Lid spasms

Point five – Field of vision:

- Check how the person sees certain horizontal points
- Amsler grid in the middle of vision
- Tangent screen
- Goldmann static or kinetic perimetry
- Automated perimetry

Point six – Slit lamp assessment on the fundus. This is to check the retina and optic nerve.

Point seven – Movement:

- Position of the head and face, slant of head
- Fixation inclination for close and far
- Fixing with the weaker or stronger eye
- More power or greater ability to see in the eye that fixes
- Rotation of the eye; grades: -4 is no ability to move, 0 is ordinary
- Monocular motility
- Block the other eye when evaluating
- Check these rotating eye actions: supraduction/elevation (to the ceiling), infraduction/depression (to the floor), abduction (away from middle), adduction (to the middle), intorsion (inward), extorsion (outward)
- The majority of elevation happens because of the superior rectus (SR) muscle. The majority of depression happens because of the inferior rectus (IR) muscle.
- Movement of both eyes at the same time in the same direction (versions)
- Binocular motility
- Ability of eyes to rotate might be superior to versions

Point eight – Accommodative amplitude for each eye:

- Deviations
- Near vision, including or not including correction
- Main position and investigative positions
- Main and next most important deviation
- Primary: fixing with the stronger eye
- Next most important: fixing with the weaker eye
- Second most important deviation is superior to the most important one
- A greater amount of nerve stimulation of a muscle to make the weaker eye fixate on the target
- Nerve stimulation of a muscle makes it so the other eye has more deviation, as such: esodeviation make it turn inward, exodeviation makes it turn outward, hyperdeviation makes it turn upward, hypodeviation makes it turn downward
- Torsion, which includes incyclotorsion or exyclotorsion

Brun's nystagmus – Big amplitude and small quickness in the direction of the lesion; big quickness and small amplitude when in the opposite direction from the lesion. This condition is caused by tumors in the cerebellum and pons, and the majority has it due to acoustic neuroma.

Extraocular Muscles

The extraocular muscles are:

- Lateral rectus – Contraction of this muscle results in abduction as its main function
- Medial rectus – Contraction of this muscle results in adduction as its main function
- Superior rectus (SR) – Main function is elevation; second most important function is adduction; third most important function is intorsion
- Inferior rectus (IR) – Main function is depression; second most important function is adduction; third most important function is extorsion
- Superior oblique – Main function is intorsion; second most important function is abduction; third most important function is depression
- Inferior oblique – Main function is extorsion; second most important function is abduction; third most important function is elevation
- Congenital downbeat nystagmus – Fleeting demonstrations occur in babies who have just been born who are actually fine. It is generally poorer in the downgaze than upgaze, and it is seen in the principal position.

Stereoacuity Testing

The important points of stereoacuity testing:

- 40 arc seconds = 20/20 vision; 60 arc seconds = 20/40 vision; 100 arc seconds = 20/200 vision.
- Titmus assessment
- Double Maddox rod assessment to check torsion
- Far and close vision assessment
- Assess main and downgaze situation
- Particularly helpful with superior oblique palsy
- May be likened to funduscopic torsion
- Saccades and pursuit, both up/down and side-to-side

- Transit time
- Amplitude
- Precision
- Rate of quickness

Upbeat nystagmus – You will see rapid phase up. It may be caused by the cerebellar structure (vermis). It may be caused by the intrinsic brainstem, in which case it could be pontomesencephalic or pontomedullary, penetrating tumors in the 4th ventricle, harm to the myelin sheath of nerve(s), or tissue death or tumor in the inside of an organ.

Motility Assessments

Cover test for tropia or manifest deviation – Ask the person to fixate on the target. (The person has to have adequate sight to do this.) Obscure an eye. Watch for a change in the uncovered eye. Take the cover off. Do the same thing on the other side. If there is no shift, it is straight. This is orthotropia. A shift suggests tropia.

Cover/uncover test for phorias or latent deviation – Look at the cover test (above) since there cannot be tropia. Ask the person to fixate on target. Obscure an eye. Quickly change it to obscure the other eye. Observe the shift in the eye that is uncovered. The latent deviation is unable to act because of fusion. This assessment makes fusional control ineffective. The latent deviation is exposed with the eye's action at the time that the cover is changed to the fellow eye.

Hirschberg's test – Used for a person that is not able to fixate on a target. Put the fixation light at 33cm. Calculate deviation of light reflex beginning at the middle of the pupil to see if there is tropia.

- Decentration of 1mm = 7° = 15 prism diopters
- Pupil edge margin = 15°
- Iris = 30°
- Limbus = 45°

Krimsky method – Also for people that cannot fixate. Put the fixation light at 33cm. Add prism in front of an eye until the position of the light reflected in the cornea is in the same place in the two eyes. This gives an approximation of the true quantitative result when getting the amount of deviation.

See-saw nystagmus – Raised and inward rotation on one eye in a half-circle, then at the same time, the opposite eye goes down and outward. It is usually caused by a suprasellar or parasellar mass.

Three-step test for hypertropia, also called Bielschowsky/Parks test:

1. Discover which is higher: left eye (LE) or right eye (RE).
2. Discover whether the left or right gaze has the worst deviation.
3. Discover whether the deviation is worse with a right head tilt (RHT) or left head tilt (LHT).

Functional visual loss – Not deriving from an organic nature, this loss of sight can relate to the loss of clarity of vision or loss of field of vision. There is not an organic lesion that may b found with an assessment. Nonphysiologic reactions are used to verify the conclusion.

Internuclear ophthalmoplegia – If young, it is generally a demyelinating problem. If not young, it is usually CVA. Think about pseudo-INA of myasthenia. The other causes are brainstem abnormal growth, carcinomatous meningitis, disease due to cancer, chiari deformity, too much cerebrospinal fluid in the skull, a disease with wasting away, drugs, brainstem dead tissue, metabolic problems, postirradiation loss of myelin sheath, bleeding in the brainstem or subdural area, or injury.

Nonorganic Visual Loss

Assessments for Nonorganic Visual Loss Include:

- Optokinetic nystagmus drum for severe loss
- Mirror evaluation for no light perception
- Testing for a sense of body positioning for severe visual loss (proprioception)
- Forced acuity
- Near vision
- Potential acuity meter
- Red-green glasses
- Three-dimensional depth (steropsis)
- Pupil reactions

Assessments for Nonorganic Faults in the Field of Vision Includes:

- Check the constricted field, as follows:
  - Tangent screen
  - Loss of vision in one eye for half of the visual field, binasal or bitemporal loss of vision for half of the visual field
  - Overlapping field from another hemifield
- Saccadic assessment

Periodic alternating nystagmus – You sill see a minute to a minute-and-a-half beats in one direction, and then it will move to the other direction. It is seen in the main position, so you have to watch any back-and-forth nystagmus to see if it changes direction. It is uniplanar.

Problems with field of vision that indicate nonorganic disease include:

- Both eyes are constricted, and they do not expand with greater distance. This is tunnel field.
- Overlapped or reversed isopters
- Coiled isopters
- Loss of vision in one eye for half of the visual field which continues with binocular assessment

Junctional visual field defects – Generally the result of a mass lesion. This may be a benign tumor in the pituitary gland, pharyngioma, aneurysm, or other. You may see a problem in the field of vision for one eye and superotemporal field problem for the opposite eye. You may see a problem in the nasal or temporal hemianopic field of vision on one side. Do an imaging study of the nervous system. If possible, use an MRI.

Visual Field Defects

Unilateral nerve fiber bundle defect – Area of lessened vision that becomes a blind spot. It is a lesion on the optic nerve or retina on one side of the body. The problem in terms of how big it is, how thick, and its form is directly related to the lesion in the optic nerve or retina. If the gap is in the middle or near the middle it is an indication of disease in the macula or optic nerve. The nerve fiber layer or retina could develop problems in both eyes. These may include glaucoma, separation in the retina, or another issue. When it is compressive, nerve fiber problems may arise so the nerves do not function properly. Be vigilant and watchful with the ophthalmoscope. Look at the optic nerve head. Issues to rule out include assessment artifacts, disease in the retina, glaucoma and optic nerve disorder.

Bilateral cecocentral or central scotomas – Although this might originate from optic nerve disorder in both eyes for any reason, other causes are seen more frequently. The cause may be lazy eye due to a toxin or nutrition problem, a problem in the optic nerve that has an outcome of disrupting the myelin in both eyes, syphilis, occipital lesions in the macula of both eyes, disease in the macula of both eyes, or Leber's optic nerve disorder (which is inherited). Make sure the problem is not a toxin such as heavy metal or ethambutol. Check for a nutrition problem. Do an imaging study of the nervous system. Check for Leber's.

Bilateral pontine lesions – the patient's eye may not be able to do any horizontal movement. Even with ongoing lesions, the reflexive actions may not be affected. Scattered lesions could result in lessened selective saccadic actions. The up and down actions might be negatively affected.

Bitemporal step or flavor visual field defect – This is a chiasmal lesion pending the establishment of another problem. Look at pseudochiasmal fields, tilted disc syndrome, defect in the structure of the eye (coloboma), disease of the nasal retina for both eyes, glaucoma, optic nerve disorder in both eyes or a lesion that influences the chiasm. These lesions may include a tumor in the pituitary gland, tumor in the meninges, craniopharyngioma, bulge in an artery in the internal carotid area, another form of tumor, injury, or a problem with the myelin in the nervous system. Carefully look at chiasm when you do an imaging study of the nervous system.

Paralytic pontine wall-eye – Unchallenged action deriving from PPRF that has no problems along with one and a half syndrome results in an eye misalignment in which one eye turns outward. This is a condition that goes along with one and a half syndrome.

Homonymous hemianopsia – Originates with retrochiasmal disease. Total homonymous hemianopsia stays in one specific area of the nervous system and will not move to another part. The lesions that correspond more in how they look, dimensions, and form are located toward the posterior. Corresponding in how they look is not a factor if the person has total hemianopsia.

Coloboma – You can see the defect with an ophthalmoscope on the optic nerve. It is caused by unfinished or abnormal shutting of the embryonic fissure. This is a problem that is present at birth. The patient may have no indications or he may have loss of visual acuity.

Downbeat nystagmus – When identifying, you will see quick phase down which is poorer with the downgaze. It is caused by a number of issues, including cervicomedullary junction lesions, alcohol, brainstem and stroke of the cerebellum, encephalitis demyelinating disease, drugs, toxins, obtained, hereditary, injury to the head, and the presence of cancer in the body.

Homonymous Hemianopsia

In order to find the place where the homonymous hemianopsia is, look at the following:

- Optic tract – look for APD on the opposite side, band wasting away in the optic disc, and homonymous hemianopsia which is, by and large, not corresponding
- Lateral geniculate body – look for incompatible wedge faults; one line of the field may not be affected
- Temporal lobe – look for a fault which is thicker in the superior of Meyer's loop; look for a "pie in the sky" gap in vision

- Parietal lobe – look for incompatible fault which will be more dense in the inferior. The problem has a higher chance of being total if there is a split in the macula. Look for right or left-sided lesions. Look for signs that the issue is occipital.

Optic Nerve Head Disorders

Coloboma – You will see the unusual optic nerve, a shiny white dug-out place on an optic disc that is bigger than normal, and the bare sclera can be seen since there is a lack of retina, pigment epithelium in the retina, and choroid which are right next to and go right along with the optic nerve. It is generally inferonasal. It may be in one or both eyes. A total scotoma will directly relate to this problem. The problem may be isolated, or it could be linked to iris coloboma, another eye irregularity or another irregularity in the body. There is no medical attention, and the problem generally does not worsen with time.

Optic pit – Present at birth, this is a fault in the optic nerve. There may be no indications, or the patient may experience lessened visual acuity or wavy and distorted vision. You may see a little dug-out place on the optic nerve rim, generally on the temporal side (but it can also be nasal or in the middle). 15% of people have it in both eyes. It could be linked to serous retinal detachment. It can go into the macula. Use fluorescein x-ray and laser procedures if there is serous detachment. Many times the serous detachment will heal on its own. Otherwise no medical attention is needed. Surgical removal of the vitreous may be done if lasers do not work. This problem can come back again.

Optic nerve hypoplasia and dysplasia – Optic nerve hypoplasia is present at birth as an optic nerve that is little. It may be caused by aplasia in very uncommon instances, or it may be due to abnormal development or underdevelopment. The patient may have no indications or lessened vision. It generally does not worsen with time. It may be 20/25 to no ability to perceive light. It is not possible to tell the acuity just by looking at the disc. There are faults in the field of vision.

You may see it in one or both eyes, with eye misalignment, involuntary and rapid eye movements, superimposed lazy eye, indications in the fundus, and a little optic disc (1/3 – ½ of a regular size). It may have pallor or not. A regular optic nerve should have these measurements: 1.38mm across and 1.46mm up-and-down. You may see the double-ring indication, wasting away in the peripapillary area, sclera/lamina cribrosa on the outside ring and a lack of RPE on the inside ring, lessened density in the nerve fiber layer and blood vessels in the retina that appear regular. Linked to this problem include indications of developmental delay (which is the most frequently seen), a problem with hypothalamic or pituitary elements, endocrine impairment, and irregularities in the face, eyes or skeleton.

Usually has no known cause, but there is a higher chance of getting it if the mother is young, ingested drugs while pregnant such as alcohol or phenytoin, had maternal diabetes, trisomy 18 or trisomy 21, intrauterine cytomegalovirus and hepatitis, or toxemia while pregnant. (Note: it is not certain whether toxemia is a risk element.) The patient will need a pediatric endocrinology assessment. Check the patient for hypothalamic hypopituitarism, neonatal hypoglycemia, diabetes insipidus, a problem with growth hormones, and thyroid hormones. Do an imaging study of the nervous system. Utilize stereo disc pictures. When the person gets old enough, test the field of vision. Medical attention includes help for endocrine disease, trying a patch for lazy eye, fixing the refractive problems, and the use of safety glasses.

Developmental abnormalities of midline brain structures (de Morsier syndrome) – these irregularities include:

- Anterior commissure does not develop properly
- Lack of the membrane that separates the lateral ventricles of the brain (septum pellucidum)
- Corpus callosum does not develop properly
- Central nervous system has an encephalocele in the area of the base of the skull

Tilted optic disc – Also called Fuchs coloboma, inferior conus or inversion/dysversion of disc. This condition is present from birth so that the optic disc is tilted. The problem may be bilateral or unilateral, and it can have an outcome of a fault in the field of vision. 80% of people have it in both eyes. There is a 3.4% incidence rate. You may see an oval disc with a smaller measurement across the disc, depression which is generally in the inferior, elevation which is generally in the superior, and crescent which is generally inferior (towards the tilt). The vessels in the retina are oblique, coming out from the superotemporal disc, moving along nasally, and then moving towards the temporal area. You may see hypopigmentation and problems in the field of vision.

Use pictures of the optic disc, check field of vision assessments, look at ectasia to see if it correlates to the place where the fault is, and do an MRI if there is a vertical step. The problem does not generally worsen with time, and there is no medical attention.

Papilledema – This word only ought to be used to describe excess swelling and fluid in the optic disc which is caused by too much intracranial pressure. Another type of puffing-up in the optic disc ought to only be discussed as an optic disc edema. There are a variety of causes for too much intracranial pressure, including uncontrolled cell growth, infection, inflammation, injury, permeation, blood vessels, bleeding in the subarachnoid area, venous sinus blood clot, too much cerebrospinal fluid in the skull, or pseudotumor cerebri.

Although the problem is generally in both eyes, some people have it in only one eye or develop an asymmetric case. The person's sight and ability to see colors is saved if the case is early. There can be temporary lessening of sight which goes on for a few seconds and causes restricted visibility. You may see swelling and fluid in the optic disc which includes excess blood in the disc, cloudy nerve fiber layer, bleeding in the peripapillary area, cotton-wool spots, venous expansion, exudates in the retina, and Paton's lines in the peripapillary area. You may find problems in the field of vision. There will not be a problem in the afferent pupil except when the case is harsh and asymmetric.

Do an imaging study of the nervous system and lumbar puncture. Medical attention includes handling the reason for the problem, acetazolamide, corticosteroids, and surgery for people that do not respond to other treatment. This may include the surgical creation of a window-like opening on the optic nerve sheath or inserting a lumboperitoneal shunt. Similar symptoms may indicate pseudopapilledema or another form of swelling and fluid in the optic disc in both eyes.

Pseudotumor cerebri – Interacranial pressure is more than it should be, but the imaging study of the nervous system is regular and the cerebrospinal fluid (CSF) is fine. The patient is generally a young female who struggles with obesity. If the person is male, not overweight, or older, be very cautious when identifying this condition.

The cause is generally not known. It is linked to a block in the venous pathway due to sagittal sinus thrombosis or a radical neck operation. It is linked to an endocrine, chemical process in the body, or bodily disease, such as a deficiency of parathyroid hormone, Addison's disease, kidney failure, systemic lupus erythematosus, or Behcet's disease. It is linked to agents from outside the body such as vitamin A, tetracycline, coming off of steroids, nalidixic acid, anabolic steroids, or lithium. The patient may experience papilledema, although this is not necessary in order to identify the condition. There may be 6th-nerve palsy that is not localized, and other than that there are not any other cranial nerves affected and there are no other indications from a focal neurological point of view. The patient may experience pain in the head, short-term (in seconds) blocks in sight, and pulsatile tinnitus.

Do an imaging study of the nervous system and a lumbar puncture. Assess the opening pressure. The person may get significant head pain which is difficult to manage and does not get better with drugs. There may be lessening of sight which worsens with time. Medical attention includes handling the linked problem appropriately, getting rid of any outside agents which may be contributing to the problem and losing weight. Drugs used include acetazolamide and corticosteroids. Other types of drugs are not as frequently used such as digoxin and furosemide. Other options include optic nerve sheath surgery to create a window-like opening or inserting a lumboperitoneal shunt. Check the patient's field of vision and take pictures of the optic disc.

Optic nerve head drusen – Calcified, glassy and translucent bodies inside the optic disc matter which can result in lessening of the visual field. It is present at birth, and some people have inherited it in an autosomal dominant way. The person generally white. Someone who is black is very unlikely to have it. It generally has no indications for the patient. There can be a gradual worsening of the field of vision. This problem is commonly in an arc-shape, a blind place in vision which gets bigger or a constriction of the field of vision. It is very uncommon to have lessened visual acuity; if the patient has this, there is probably another problem as well. There can be temporary blocks in vision.

Linked to other problems including retinitis pigmentosa, pseudoxanthoma elasticum, angioid streaks, bleeding in the retina, folds in the choroid and retina and migraine headaches. 66% of people have it in both eyes. You may see scattered and shapeless deposits on the optic nerve which are nasal the majority of the time (as opposed to temporal), no cup, a little disc and an unusual network of blood vessels in the disc. There is a lack of exudates and a lack of enlarged blood vessels in the disc. The problem is inclined to be more obvious as the person gets older. If the patient is a child, the disc drusen is buried. You may see too many blood vessels in the subfovea and drusen transilluminate inside of the disc head. The patient will need a clinical identification of the problem. Other people in the family should be checked.

Optic nerve head drusen – To find buried drusen, do an ultrasound on the nerve head. A CT scan is only for very unusual cases to identify calcified drusen. Use preinjection fluorescein angiography to identify an impediment of filling in the peripapillary choroid and self-induced fluorescence (not useful for buried drusen). Take pictures of the stereo disc. Similar symptoms may indicate arteritic optic nerve that is not getting enough blood flow and not functioning normally, an artery block in the retina, vein block in the retina, subretinal neovascular membrane, and subretinal exudation or heme.

Melanocytoma – Present at birth; pigmented irregularity on the optic disc head which generally has no patient indications. You may see a lesion is black and can be a little bit raised. No assessments or medical attention. It may get gradually bigger. Similar symptoms may indicate melanoma or hamartoma which is both in the retina and RPE.

Myelinated nerve fiber layer – Although the process of creating a myelin sheath regularly ends at the lamina cribosa, it can arise on the retina's nerve fiber layer. This problem is present at birth and generally has no patient indications. A clinical identification of the problem is needed. It stays the same throughout time. No medical attention is used. Similar symptoms may indicate cotton-wood patch, infiltrates on the retina or a small artery block.

Ischemic optic neuropathy (ION) – Clinical collection of symptoms that is marked with significant lessening of sight, proof of abnormal optic nerve functioning, and in most cases an inflamed optic nerve if the patient is aged. The cause may be arteritic ION and giant cell inflammation of arteries, or it may be nonarteritic ION with another abnormal vascular problem such as diabetes or hardened arteries.

If the case is nonarteritic, the patient may experience significant lessened sight and/or field of vision that is generally an altitudinal problem, a problem with color vision, the condition in one eye and no pain. If the condition is arteritic, it generally has worse lessening of sight, can be in both eyes and may also have issues in the whole body such as head pain, pain in the jaw, sore scalp, general and nonspecific discomfort, high body temperature, lower body weight than normal, or no appetite and severe weight loss. The person is generally over 40 years old. GCA is seen in people over 55. People commonly are seen with vasculopathic issues which increase the hazard.

You will generally see an inflamed optic nerve in the anterior. If the condition is only in one eye or if it is in both eyes but not evenly balanced, you may see a comparative afferent fault in the pupil. There is no flare-up in the anterior or posterior segment. Check the erythrocyte sedimentation rate (ESR). Do C-reactive protein assessment to check for giant cell arteritis. A tissue sample to look at the temporal artery may be done to check for GCA as well. When doing the biopsy, look for the superficial temporal artery down in the skin and subcutaneous tissue and on the surface of the temporalis fascia. This condition will have swelling in the temporal artery. There may be GCA or not. The internal elastic lamina is not normal and there are too many cells in the innermost layer.

If the case is nonarteritic, the patient will commonly have lessened ability to see that stays the same, but it could unexpectedly get better or there could be worsening as time goes by. It is influenced by a little cup-to-disc ratio. If the case is arteritic there is commonly significant loss of sight. If no medical attention is found, there will be significant loss of sight in both eyes. Similar symptoms may indicate abnormal optic nerve functions with infection, infiltration, compression, toxin, or inflammation. It may also indicate an abnormal optic nerve function that is inherited, such as Leber's optic neuropathy.

Medical attention for nonarteritic cases includes tending to the vasculopathic danger elements that the person may have and one aspirin every day to lessen the danger for the other eye. optic nerve sheath decompression is not used. Check-ups should be done when they are needed. If the case is arteritic, use prednisone taken by mouth and think about steroids put into the vein if there is significant loss of sight. 65% of people will get arteric ION in the other eye if no medical attention is sought. Track the ESR and clinical indications, and make sure the patient goes off of steroids gradually.

Optic neuritis – This expression refers to any abnormal optic nerve function that occurs with no known cause (for the majority of cases) or disrupts the myelin coating of the nervous system structures (such as with multiple sclerosis). The problem may also be due to an infection from a virus, syphilis, catch scratch disease, Lyme disease or other type of infection. It may be due to a flare-up from collagen vascular disease, sarcoid, or other inflammation. Although the person is generally a young grown person, this condition may arise in any stage of life. The person is more commonly a woman, but it does arise for men as well.

A common case will be marked with significant loss of sight in one eye and hurting that gets worse when the eye moves around. Uncommon indications include the problem beginning in both eyes at the same time for a grown person, flare-up in the anterior or posterior segment, star formation in the macula, no hurting, no real getting better, and prior problems with flare-up or infections. You may see lessened ability to see or lessened visual field, comparative afferent fault in the pupil if the case is in one eye or in two, unbalanced eyes and a lack of eye inflammation in the anterior and posterior. 65% of people have regular optic nerve, but 35% have inflammation in the optic nerve.

90% of people will be able to get back to the vision that they had before. If the case is typical, only an MRI is needed to see if there is demyelination. If the problem is not typical, include lab tests as well, which will be contingent upon what is discovered during examination. When the MRI is fine, just watch the patient to see if it gets better. Steroids into a vein may be used. If the case is not typical, think about steroids in the vein and think about doing more assessments to check for MS. The patient will need to be checked during the 4 to 6 weeks after the onset to make sure it is getting better. Watch this patient for MS. Similar symptoms may indicate ION or abnormal optic nerve functioning due to inflammation, infection, compression, toxin, inherited factors or infiltration.

Optic Nerve and Chiasm Disorders

Toxic or nutritional optic neuropathy – The person will generally show the problem as balanced in both eyes with gradual lessening of sight over time. The patient may experience a fault in the field of vision and lessened visual acuity. At first, the optic nerve will look fine, but wasting away will occur as the problem progresses. The cause is either a nutritional insufficiency or a toxin. Do an MRI on the head, check for vitamin B_{12}, and check for folate and the complete blood count. You only need to do a urine test for heavy metals when the case indicates that it is necessary.

Marcus-Gunn jaw wink – Irregular rising of the lid including action in the jaw; due to problem that is present at birth where one involuntary action (in jaw muscles) goes with a voluntary one (in levator). It is an abnormal neural link. The patient generally has droopy eyelids from birth. A clinical identification of the problem is needed, and there is no medical attention.

Leber's hereditary optic neuropathy – Very uncommon and hereditary condition mitochondrial abnormal optic nerve function. It is seen in young adult males who are generally in the second decade of life for the majority of cases, but it can be seen in women as well. The patient may experience lessened visual acuity which is significant, quick, ceaseless, and does not hurt. It generally is 20/200 to the hand motion range, although 20/20 to no light perception has been seen. There is lessened field of vision with middle or cecocentral blind spots. Both eyes are affected, with the second one getting the condition within days, weeks or months following the first. 40% - 50% of people get it in both eyes at the same time.

When lessened sight occurs, observations may be found on the fundus. There are three fundus warnings:

- Enlarged small blood vessel disease in abnormal optic nerve function
- Visible inflammation in the nerve fiber layer near the disc
- Fluorescein blood vessel x-ray commonly lets you see pseudoedema; seeping from the disc is only shown in very uncommon instances

Following the loss of sight, the fundus will have weakened arterioles, lessened nerve fiber layer, particularly in the papillomacular bundle, and there can be nonglaucomatous cupping. Although the majority of people will not generally have another problem in the body, some people have another linked problem. There are sometimes heart conduction problems. Some people have dystonia or another form of minor neurological problem. Make sure it is not another form of abnormal optic nerve function. The main problem is mitochondrian DNA fault. Medical attention includes lessening chemical function stress in the optic nerve. This means that the person should stop smoking, using toxins which are problems with optic nerves or lessening injury if possible. The medical attention used is not established, but does include multivitamins, folate, vitamin B_{12}, thiamine, and idebenone and other coenzyme Q10 analogues. A number of people will unexpectedly get better, but the majority of patients do not experience this and have a static condition instead.

Oculopharyngeal muscular dystrophy - Hereditary (autosomal dominant) paralysis of eye muscles; generally of French-Canadian descent; 40 years old. You may see autosomal recessive or random instances in people of another descent. The person will experience a hard time swallowing, ophthalmoplegia which ranges in severity, orbicularis muscles that are not strong, and temporalis degeneration. Clinically identify the problem, and use a tissue sample of the muscle to study irregularities. No medical attention.

These Are Toxic to the Optic Nerve:

Amantadine, amiodarone, amoproxan, aniline dyes, barbiturates, cafergot, cabromal, carbon disulfide, carbon tetrachloride, cephaloridine, chloramphenicol, chlorodinitrobenzene, clioquinol, dichlorodiphenyltrichloroethane (DDT), digitalis, dinitrotoluene, disulfiram (antabuse), d-penicillamine, diiodohydroxyquin, elcatonin, emetine, ethambutol, ethylchlorvinol (placidyl), ethylene glycol, 5-fluorouracil, glue sniffing, halogenated hydroxyquinolone, heavy metals, hexachlorophene, iodoform, iodopyracet (diodrast), isoniazid, Lysol, methanol, methyl acetate, methyl bromide, octamoxin, organophosphate pesticides, penicillamine, phenazone (antipyren), pheniprazine (catron), plasmocid, quinine, sodium fluoride, streptomycin, styrene (vinyl benzyl), sulfonamides, thallium, thioglycolates, tolbutamide (orinase), trichloroethylene, vincristine.

These May Cause a Nutritional Lack in the Optic Nerve:

Pernicious anemia, nutritional insufficiency (such as from a vegan diet or too much alcohol), lack of vitamin B_{12}, folate.

Infiltrative or inflammatory optic neuropathy - This problem can imitate optic neuritis which is demyelinating or of no known cause. The patient may experience loss of visual acuity and lessened ability to see colors. You may see it in one or both eyes with an afferent fault in the pupil, pallor or inflammation of the optic disc, or an optic disc that looks regular (retrobulbar). Unusual things you may see include the condition beginning at the same time in both eyes, no hurting, a condition that will not get better, flare-up in the anterior or posterior segment, worsening with time, repeated instances of the problem, and a steroid reaction or a steroid reliant case.

Infiltrative or inflammatory optic neuropathy - may be caused by unusual and uncontrolled cell growth as in the case of cancer in the plasma cells, carcinomatous meningitis, leukemia, or cancer in the lymph nodes. It may be caused by paraneoplastic problems. It may be caused by an infection from cryptococcal meningitis, aspergillus, TB or syphilis. It may be due to an inflammatory problem in the body such as contiguous sinus disease, sarcoidosis, lupus erythematosus in the body, or a flare-up of bowel disease. Do an MRI to look at the head and orbit (when needed), CBC, assessment for syphilis, assessment for antinuclear antibodies, chest x-ray, angiotensin-converting enzyme, lysozyme, lumbar puncture, gallium scan when sarcoidosis may be present, PPD skin assessment if TB could be present, and anti-dsDNA assessments when lupus erythematosus in the body could be present.

Optic Pathway Tumors

Optic gliomas – One of the two frequently seen forms of optic pathway tumors. (The other is meningiomas.) These glial tumors can create an issue in the optic nerve, chiasm, or tract. It is mainly seen in kids and young, fully grown people (both male and female), but it may arise in any stage of life. It is linked to neurofibromatosis type 1. The frequency is very uncommon. It accounts for 1% - 2% of tumors found in the orbit, 2% of new tumors within the cranial cavity, and 3% - 6% of tumors in the cranial cavity for children. It may be in one or both eyes.

As the tumor is closer to the anterior, the patient has a better prediction for the future. The mortality rate is contingent upon where it is found. If it is only in the optic nerve, it is 14%. If it is in the chiasm, it is around the range of 47%. If there is hypothalamic participation, it is 91%. No pain. The gradual worsening of vision over time includes 87% lessening of general sight, 26% with sight that is 20/20 to 20/40, 19% of sight that is 20/50 to 20/200, and 55% of sight that is 20/300 or worse.

Localization of lesion: may be brainstem, subarachnoid area, cavernous sinus, orbit, neuromuscular junction, a number of extraocular muscles, or it may be a multifocal disease which is influenced by any of these joined together. Do an imaging study of the nervous system and any other necessary assessments to find out where the problem is. Check for myasthenia gravis.

If the patient has hypothalamic indications or indications of endocrine involvement, the person will have diabetes insipidus, diencephalic debilitation, abnormally early puberty, sleepiness, and abnormally poor pattern of growth. There may be problems in the field of vision. You will see irregular protuberance of the eyeball from its socket, inflammation or wasting away in the disc, eye misalignment, and rapid and involuntary eye movements. Glioma should be looked for in a child that has inexplicable loss of sight, nystagmus in one eye or in both eyes but unbalanced between the two, wasting away in the optic area, hypothalamic indications, diencephalic indications, spasmus nutans, see-saw nystagmus, or too much cerebrospinal fluid in the skull. Image study of the nervous system. A CT is likely to be insufficient. Do MRI. Look for traits of neurofibromatosis. Check the patient's growth. Look for signs of early puberty. Assess the person's family. There is not usually a need for biopsy when it is obviously in the chiasm or nerve, intraxial, or if there is a record of NF type 1. The person may need a biopsy if the indications are irregular or if there is penetration or compression of the chiasm. Similar symptoms may indicate parenchymal optic nerve enlargement or extraparenchymal indications. Medical attention is debatable and unproven.

Traumatic optic neuropathy – imaging study of the nervous system. Medical attention includes a variety of corticosteroid options, dexamethasone, methylprednisolone, two days of steroids and then an oral taper of prednisone. If the steroids do not work or if the person on prednisone experiences continued loss of sight, use surgical decompression of the optic canal. Surgery options include canthotomy, cantholysis, a drain of the hematoma, and decompression.

Meningiomas of the anterior visual pathway – Benign spreading in the meningeal sheath into the optic nerve resulting in putting stress on other structures. It is frequently seen in the middle of life, mainly around the 50's. It is more common in women and white people. It does not hurt. The person will experience a slow lessening of sight, problems in the field of vision, alteration in mental ability (when frontal), double vision when it affects the cavernous sinus area, and the loss of the sense of smell when it affects the olfactory groove.

Superior oblique myokymia – On and off actions of the SOM with an outcome of double vision that comes and goes or swinging vision. The cause is not known, but could be due to injury or it may arise after fourth-nerve palsy. It does not generally get linked to problems in the intracranial area.

Use a slit lamp, and do MRI when there are indications of problems in the intracranial area. Use patches, drugs, or a strabismus operation.

Meningiomas of the anterior visual pathway – You may see wasting away in the optic area and/or swelling and fluid in the disc. You may find optociliary shunt vessel. Do an imaging study of the nervous system, usually in the form of an MRI. Utilize a CT to look for hyperostotic bone. Medical attention includes removing it with neurosurgery. It usually does not respond to radiation or chemotherapy.

Traumatic optic neuropathy (TON) – Clinically identified problem that is marked with a prior record of collision to the head, face or orbit. Most probably the harm then moves in a circuitous or non-circuitous manner into the optic nerve with an outcome of a range of lessened sight. Injury to the head, face, forehead or orbit, and could be resulting from pressure, a non-circuitous collision, bleeding in the retrobulbar area, too much pressure inside the orbit, blood clot or fluid in the subperiosteal or intrasheath area, a bruising injury, fluid and swelling or inflammation in the optic nerve, harm to the vascular area, or swelling. The patient may experience lessened sight from 20/20 to no ability to see light, and he may have lessened ability in the visual field. You may find a relative afferent fault in the pupil of one or both eyes, wasting away in the optic area as time passes and inflammation in the optic nerve in some cases.

Brown syndrome – Restricted rise during adduction due to an irregularity of the superior oblique tendon sheath complex. It may be present at birth or obtained due to an injury or inflammation of the tendon sheaths. There is no medical attention. When identifying the problem, the forced rotations of the eye will be positive.

Palsies, Illusions, and Hallucinations

Visual illusions and hallucinations – Problems with perception of the area around may be due to irregular data gathering of visual cues which go away when the eyes are shut in the case of illusions. For a hallucination, visual cues are not involved.

Visual illusions – May be caused by a lens with a deviation in shape, double convex lens irregularity, a tint in a shade of yellow/brown, a condition after having a cataract taken out in which everything looks blue, an irregularity in sight in which everything is a shade of red, a variation in the tear film or cornea, variations in the indexes of refraction, or a disease in the retina. The patient may experience a problem with processing information in terms of the form and dimensions, location, how far away something is, how it is moving, or too many images. Medical attention includes antiepileptic drugs or anticonvulsants.

Hallucinations – The patient may experience lessened sight and abrasions in the anterior sight corridor, abrasions in the sight and temporal cortex ahead, problems in the brainstem limbic circuits, and migraine. These may be caused by a seizure in only one part of the brain, irregularity in the CNS neurotransmitters, inability to suppress a state of dreaming (as in not being fully conscious or having sight deficiency), development of the problem not related to anything else, abnormality of the vestibule apparatus, or an agent that has an effect on the mind. Comfort the person, remove any drugs that could be causing the problem, determine if the problem is an illusion or a hallucination, determine that migraine is not the issue, and when the case necessitates, use and MRI and EEG.

Fourth-nerve palsies – Medical attention includes a patch, prism, and strabismus operation when there is a static variation. Similar symptoms may indicate myasthenia gravis, pseudotumor in the orbit, tumor in the orbit, thyroid eye disease, or skew.

Double vision (up and down) in one eye, a deviating head posture, double vision that is worse when looking down, subjective torsion (or none in some cases), incidences that are present at birth, big vertical fusional amplitudes and venerable HT. It can arise in any stage of life in both males and females. Double vision (up and down) is worse when looking down, hypertropia on one side, superior oblique lessened ability, subjective excyclotorsion when utilizing double Maddox rod, and observable excyclotorsion when utilizing fundoscope. If the problem is not by itself, do an MRI, lumbar puncture, GCA if the person is aged, and think about myasthenia gravis. If the problem is by itself and the patient is a kid, it may have been present at birth, so look at old pictures for indications. Think about doing an MRI. Identification of the problem will be contingent upon past medical accounts and assessments. If the problem was present at birth or caused by injury, nothing else is needed. A vasculopathic case will be 6-8 weeks, and you should watch closely and use medical attention for any danger signs. An imaging test of the nervous system may be used. If the problem is not vasculopathic, do MRI, lumbar puncture (to check for meningeal indications), assessments of vasculopathic indications, and think about myasthenia gravis.

Third-nerve palsies – You will find the third-nerve nucleus in the midbrain. It is made up of a number of subnuclei. These act to help the inferior rectus, inferior oblique, medial rectus on the same side of the body, levator (which is helped with one nucleus in the middle), and superior rectus on the other side. Fibers in the pupil come from the Edinger-Westphal nuclei. The cluster of third nerve goes by vital things in the midbrain and goes into the subarachnoid area. From there it goes into the lateral wall in the cavernous sinus. Then it goes into the orbit by way of the superior orbital fissure. From there is splits into superior and inferior.

Sixth-nerve palsies – Double vision (up and down) and in one eye and worse when looking towards the paretic side. It happens at any time of life in both males and females. You may see constructed or lagging abduction, unusual way of turning the face to achieve fusion, and vertical abnormality in some cases. If the case is not alone, do MRI, lumbar puncture, GCA for an aged person, and think about myasthenia gravis. If it is alone and the person is in childhood, think about sixth-nerve pareses following a virus, MRI, and assessments as needed. If it is vasculopathic, watch for 6-8 weeks, assess vasculopatic issues, make sure it is not GCA for an aged person, and consider an imaging study of the nervous system. If it is not vasculopathic, do MRI, lumbar puncture, assess for vasculopathic issues, and think about myasthenia gravis. Kids may need lazy eye medical attention. Utilize patch or prism, and if the alteration is static, a strabismus operation can be done.

Localization of lesion including a number of cranial nerve palsies – The problem may be in the brainstem, subarachnoid area, cavernous sinus, orbit, neuromuscular junction, a number of extraocular muscles, or it may be a multifocal disease which is influenced by any of these joined together. Do imaging study of the nervous system and any other necessary assessments to find out where the problem is. Check for myasthenia gravis if the person has no hurting and the pupil is not affected but there is nonproptotic paralysis of eye muscles.

Facial nerve palsy – Supranuclear syndrome is caused by an abrasion in the frontal cortex and creates limitations in the hand, tongue, or top extremity areas. There is nerve stimulation on both sides to muscles of the brows and orbicularis muscles and nerve stimulation on the opposite side affecting the bottom 2/3 of the face. With nuclear or cerebellopontine angle syndrome, the problem is damage to the myelin sheath of nerve(s), new/uncontrolled cell growth, tissue death, or bleeding. The patient may experience complete weakness on the face on one side, lessened ability for tearing, abnormal sensitivity to sounds and lessened ability to taste on the anterior 2/3 of the tongue. Gradenigo syndrome happens because of inflammation of the mastoid or middle ear, and results in abnormality of the cranial nerves including nerves V (causing hurting face), VI, and VII. Geniculate ganglionitis may be an indication, and there may be more superficial petrosal nerve. Do an MRI of the 7th nerve and other testing as necessary. Look for Bell's palsy if the condition is alone. Moisturize the eyes, do lateral tarsorrhaphy when there is exposure keratopathy, and use a gold weight in the top eyelid.

Cavernous Sinus Syndrome and THS

Medical attention should be done on the reason for the problem. For THS, use steroids, but make sure it is not an infection first. Similar symptoms indicate neoplastic, vascular, infection, flare-up, of no known cause, or injury issues. Inside the cavernous sinus you will find the eye motor nerves of the cranium, parts of trigeminal nerve, the inside carotid artery, and the eye sympathetic nerves. Since these are present, abrasions in this area can create problems with them. If the lesion goes into the anterior, abnormal optic nerve functioning, proptosis, or other problems may occur. THS is of no known cause, and is a flare-up with paralysis of the muscles with hurting. It is found in the cavernous sinus. THS is only identified by making sure it is not one of a number of other problems first. These are found in both men and women, with the 50's being a frequently seen age (but may be 35 to 75). The patient will experience hurting, nerve problems, 22% do have an affected pupil, 4% have Horner syndrome, and optic nerve problems are not frequently seen. Do an imaging study such as MRI, lumbar puncture when needed, and lab tests as needed.

Chronic Progressive External Ophthalmoplegia

Chronic progressive external ophthalmoplegia (CPEO) is not definitely defined in terms of what causes it. Progressive muscle weakness (myopathy) problems are not usually in regards to the muscles of the eyes. CPEO types are as follows:

- Worsening with time paralysis of eye muscle(s), including CPEO that is alone, Kearns-Sayre syndrome, oculopharyngeal abnormal development of muscles, myotonic abnormal development of muscles, and oculopharyngeal myopathy that is alone.
- Differentiate from stable paralysis of eye muscle problems
- Another form of eye muscle weakness that gets worse with time
- Linked to neurodegenerative disease
- Presumed mitochondrial syndrome, including progressive muscle weakness in the face, bulbar or limb areas, ataxia, spasticity, and abnormal development of peripheral nerves, no ability to hear, dementia, wasting away of the optic nerve, wasting away of the pigment of the retina, irregular heart conduction, and irregularities of the endocrine system, skin or skeleton
- Stephens syndrome

Kearns-Sayre Syndrome

Kearns-Sayre syndrome begins before age 20 and can arise in babyhood, but not congenital. Paralysis of eye muscles begins following the fifth birthday. Other family members will not usually have it, but it could be autosomal dominant. The majority are random. The problem gradually worsens and affects the horizontal and vertical muscles. In the beginning, the muscles to look down may not be affected. Double vision is not generally seen. Early on, you will see ptosis (not every case) and problems in both eyes (but not balanced). People utilize the eyebrows to raise the lids. There can be complete paralysis of eye muscles and it can affect the orbicularis muscle. The pupils are not affected. Sight is generally fine, but central sight may be lessened as time goes by. In unusual cases there is a pigment disease of the retina. Use coenzyme Q10 and do an operation to fix the ptosis if needed, but be careful due to the paralysis and the fact that there is no Bell's reflex.

Myotonic Dystrophy

Myotonic dystrophy is a broad problem in the muscles marked with myotonia. You may see orbicularis muscle that is not strong, difficulty relaxing muscles when shutting the lid, droopy lids, problems with eccentric gaze holding, slow ability to make the eye move from one point to another, lazy and myotic pupils, inflamed lids, dry eyes, low intraocular pressure, lens issues (polychromatic cataract, cortex star in the posterior, posterior subcapsular), alterations in the pigment of the macula, restricted field of vision, bleeding on the iris tufts, and on-and-off lid lag. Make sure it is not myasthenia gravis. Think about whether the person needs a body check-up. Check lactate and muscle tissue, do EMG, CSF, and check alterations in mitochondrial DNA. Other problems in the body may include no hair in the front of the head, wasting away in the testicles, heart irregularities, and constricted hatchet facies.

Duane Syndrome

Duane syndrome involves irregularities in abduction or adduction; linked to cocontraction in the muscles just outside the eyeball. The globe retracts and the space between the margins of the eyelids constricts. Present at birth, it is a lack of a sixth-nerve nucleus. There is also irregular nerve stimulation. The three forms include:

- Abduction – lack of retraction of globe with abduction
- Adduction – lack of retraction of globe with adduction
- Combined – lack in both

This may be in both eyes. Generally, there is no medical attention. The patient will need clinical identification of the problem.

Aberrant Regeneration

Aberrant regeneration is re-formation of the third nerve can happen with irregular nerve stimulation. It could be primary, with no prior problem with third-nerve palsy, or secondary. This does not happen when the third-nerve palsy is due to low blood flow/oxygen. The lid will be raised when the eye is raised or during adduction. The pupil is restricted during adduction, raising, or lowering. There may be any number of combinations of irregular nerve stimulation.

Supranuclear Motility Disturbances

Saccades – Quick actions to relocate the eyes and keep the target on the fovea. Problems that occur include irregularly slow, inexact or lack. If there is saratic paresis, the patient may experience a lesion, either in both eyes or in one eye (in the front). If the problem is saccades that are inexact, it could be a quick and uncontrolled action, paired action, a flutter that goes across, an action that continues while asleep, or multivectoral. If it is too slow, it could be an over or under-shoot of the target. Smoothness of saccades is desired, and if this is lacking or slow, it may be due to medications or a neurodegenerative disease. Indications of smoothness problems include a vague cogwheel pursuit and Balint syndrome. Balint syndrome includes not being able to view one thing when you want to, not being able to locate and categorize things, simultagnosia, the ability to see just one target at one time and the inability to view the whole area.

Internuclear ophthalmoplegia – Inside the pons is the end of the shared trail for horizontal saccades and pursuit. Abrasions there can affect the parapontine reticular development or sixth-nerve nucleus. This would result in an irregularity in the horizontal saccades and pursuit. The interneurons beginning at the sixth-nerve nucleus go into the medial longitudinal fasciculus on the other side. These could be harmed with an outcome of INO. Indications:

- One-sided, back-and-forth gaze palsy
- With a rostral abrasion, no problem with the vistibuloocular reflex
- With a significant abrasion, eyes that have contralateral irregularities

The patient may experience no ability to adduct, slight problem with adduction and irregular adduction on the other side. When the problem is in the midbrain, there may be rostral disease and convergence. This is known as Cogan's anterior INO. The title of the problem goes by the side of the adduction problem. When there is abrasion that is caudal, the convergence may be fine.

One and a half syndrome – This is both an abrasion of PPRF or sixth-nerve nucleus (resulting in one side having horizontal gaze palsy) and INO abrasion; both are located on the same side. This is caused by lack of blood flow to the brainstem, MS, tumor, bleeding in pons, or injury.

Midbrain lesions – When the person has vertical gaze palsy and the rostral interstitial nucleus of the MLF midbrain-thalamic intersection will be affected. When there is weakness for the downgaze, it may be caused by stroke, lesions on both sides of the dorsomedial red nucleus, Huntington's disease, PSP, or thalamic bleed. When the person has some paralysis with the upgaze, the posterior juncture will be affected, the upward saccade fibers will go into the posterior juncture, and the upgaze/downgaze fibers are separated. A vertical gaze palsy may be due to scattered wasting away procedures, gradually worsening supranuclear palsy, dead tissue, wasting away of the cortical basal area, Whipple's disease, Parkinson's disease, MS, Fisher syndrome, syphilis, Brucella group infection, tetanus, viral infection in the brain, neurofibromatosis, tuberculoma, surgery on the nervous system or injury.

Parinaud's dorsal midbrain syndrome – Marked with many discoveries, some of which are convergence-retraction rapid and involuntary eye movements, upgaze partial paralysis, and light-near dissociation which happens in the pupils. Some other frequently seen indications are lessened ability of saccades when looking up, dilated pupils, swelling around the optic nerve, a block and too much cerebrospinal fluid in the skull, and convergence spasm or paresis. Some findings that are not as frequently seen include skew variation, fourth-nerve palsy, pulled-back lid, lessened ability in upgaze, random convergence retraction actions, downbeat rapid and involuntary eye movements, unequal pupil size, accommodative spasm when looking up, actions like a serpent when looking up, and ptosis in some cases. Uncommonly seen conditions include peduncular hallucinosis, puberty that is uncommonly early, pseudoabducens palsy, too much cerebrospinal fluid in the skull, A or V pattern of eyes that turns out, and square-wave jerks. Do MRI and make sure it is not another reason. Parinaud's dorsal midbrain syndrome may be caused by tumors in the pineal gland, a germ cell tumor in the brain (usually in adolescent male), a tumor made up of several different types of tissue, brain cancer, cancer that has spread from another place in the body, too much cerebrospinal fluid in the skull, penetrating tumor into the third ventricle, pituitary stroke, a metabolic problem, syphilis in the central nervous system, another form of encephalitis, Whipple's disease, TB, certain drugs, demyelination, injury, surgery on the brain, spinal cord, or nerves, a vascular problem, or a form of degeneration.

Nystagmus

Nystagmus is quick, repeated and unusual motions in one or both eyes; may be in both eyes and unbalanced. It could be regularly back and forth or be more erratic. It could happen only in the main gaze, or it only in certain gaze activities. Some people have a mixture. Some have it from birth; others obtain it. When it is related to the functions of the body, there is an end point or end gaze, twitching nystagmus, and it is revolving. Do a caloric test to assess the vestibular and oculomotor nerve reflexes. When local, it is internuclear muscle paralysis in the external ocular area. This form has abduction nystagmus on the opposite side from the lesion, and the adduction muscles are not strong on the same side. It is in the region of the ipsilateral MLF. Nystagmus occurs in younger people with MS and older people with stroke. A muscular debility may result in pseudo INO. Another form of lesion in the brainstem may also cause this condition.

Congenital nystagmus – this form can be split into two forms, sensory and motor. This split aids in determining good clinical choices for the patient. The problem generally will not arise prior to the tenth week of life, but it is generally identified during babyhood. Some patients will not show signs until a few months have passed. If it is sensory, there is no cortical lessening of vision and the baby's sight will be 20/200 or worse. Do an imaging study of the nervous system such as MRI, do ERG, lab assessments as needed for bodily problems, and think about doing a tissue sample study of conjunctiva. Look for the eyes to move inward for focusing on a near object, lack of chaotic eye movements, null zone, a gaze location which is unfaltering when nystagmus is horizontal, balanced amplitude and quickness for the two eyes, near vision that is good, inverted pursuit and saccadic systems, a turned head to get to the null point, no problem when sleeping, and latent nystagmus.

Spasmus nutans – Obtained nystagmus during babyhood (4 months to 14 months); generally not dangerous; can be linked to glioma in the eyes. The majority will get better by 5 years old. You may see it in both eyes, but not balanced, or it may be only in one eye. There will be delicate shimmering back-and-forth action, or it may be roundabout or up-and-down. It has little amplitude and big quickness. It could go before nodding the head, and be continuous or discontinuous. Think about doing MRI on the head to look at anterior paths of sight.

Acquired binocular pendular nystagmus – Balanced amplitude each way, in a pendulum-like motion; up-and-down or side-to-side. Look at whether it was present at birth, make sure it is not caused by drugs or toxins, do imaging study of the nervous system, and use noncircuitous imaging on particular locations depending on the case. This may be due to irregular myelin functioning, oculopalatal muscle jerking, mitochondrial cell disorder, chiasm lesions, brainstem/cerebellum stroke or tumor, or Whipple's disease.

Pupil Abnormalities

Marcus-Gunn pupil – This is an afferent pupil fault. Check it with the back-and-forth flashlight assessment. A regular reaction will have pupil constriction on the same side and on the other side. Irregular reactions are as follows:

- Type I – instantaneous pupil enlargement 4+ APD
- Type II – not as quick, but clear pupil enlargement 3+ APD
- Type III – stays the same at first, then enlarges 1 – 2+ APD
- Type IV – at first becomes enlarges, then changes to become even bigger at a faster pace than the other eye, slight APD

The condition may be due to a problem in the optic nerve, significant disease in the retina or abrasion on the optic tract. It is very uncommonly due to lazy eye or bleeding in the vitreous. Sometimes it arises in the opposite side from the pretectal lesion and there is no loss of sight. Check the optic nerves and look for disease in the retina. APD with no explanation may be due to optic nerve issues.

Anisocoria – Look at how the pupil responds to light. This condition happens in around 20% of normal people, the way the lid is positioned is regular, and there is a lack of pupil enlargement. The dimension of the pupil could be different each day, anisocoria is the same whether it is light or dark and there is generally 1mm or smaller unequal pupil size. Cocaine assessment is negative. Similar symptoms may indicate body function issues, Horner syndrome, or sympathetic overaction.

Horner syndrome – Patient will have a regular light and near response, slight droopy eyelids, medium amount of constricted pupil on one side, observable sinking of the eye into the socket, upside-down droopy lower lid, inability to sweat on the face and neck, and different colors in the iris (generally if the case is present at birth). Do MRI on the middle neuron, intermediate image testing on the anterior mass of nervous tissues and imaging on the posterior mass of nervous tissues when needed.

Tonic pupil – This form of pupil will not respond to light well. There is a tonic near response. 70% if cases are in young females from 20-40 years old, with the mean being 32 years old. 4.7 out of 100,000 people have it and 10%-20% in both eyes. 20% of instances have no indications for the patient. The others have fuzzy sight, a hard time reading, light sensitivity, intense shine, ciliary twinge or brow pain when using near vision for some people and accommodation brings on a distorted curve of the cornea. Use a slit lamp to look for locations of palsy and worm-like actions. In the pupil, look at the tonic condition, how the pupil enlarges following accommodation, abnormal enlargement, or pupils that become more constricted as time goes by. Drug assessment with a small amount of pilocarpine (1/8%) may be used to see cholinergic denervation supersensitivity and a constraint of Adie's tonic pupil. A pupil with no problems will not tighten with this small amount of the drug.

Medical attention includes ESR if the person is old, which is very uncommon and assessment for syphilis. Use tinted glasses and low pilocarpine to help intense shine. Use anticholinergic (not strong) for ciliary tremor. Bifocals may be used for accommodation issues. The majority of people do not need medical attention. In terms of progression, most people will not gain back the pupil and light response, and the pupil can get progressively smaller. The majority of indications get better, but the person might stay hyporeflexic. A maximum of 4% of instances each year will progress to both eyes. Similar symptoms may indicate an infection, injury, tumor, reaction to medical attention, diabetes, nerve disorder, GCA, flare-up, amyloid, disruption in the autonomic nervous system, ongoing problems with alcohol, Guillain-Barre (Fisher type), inherited motor sensory nerve disorder (type 1 and 2) and drug obstruction.

Third-nerve palsy – In the intensive care environment having to do with the nervous system, a lone enlarged pupil gives a warning indication of third-nerve problems, like uncal herniation as an example. When the person an outpatient, one enlarged pupil which with no droopy eyelids an no problem with movement is very unlikely to indicate a problem with the third-nerve. When assessing an enlarged pupil in isolation, make sure it is not another issue making the enlarged pupil. These more frequently seen issues include tonic pupil, enlargement due to drugs, or harm in the iris. An alteration in the form of the iris could have an outcome of unequal pupil size. To identify this use a slit-lamp assessment and get a good medical history. The cause of third-nerve palsy may be a sphincter rip, old transillumination issue, proof for old or fresh flare-up, adhesion of the pupil to the lens, prior operation inside the eye, not enough oxygen in the iris, or wasting away in the iris.

Pharmacologic dilation – Generally identified with medical records and assessment. Use topical pilocarpine 1% to verify this condition. Watch out for people that may use dilating drops, such as someone who works in the health industry or someone who has been to the hospital in the near past. Look for medium to fully dilated and fixed pupil. Look for conjunctival blanching in one eye when utilizing neosynephrine. The cause could be unintentional contact with a topical agent that dilates the pupil, artificial utilization of an agent that dilates the pupil which was done on purpose, or contact with certain foliage, such as moonflower or jimsonweed.

Multiple sclerosis – The forms of multiple sclerosis include clinically proved, clinically likely, and likely. There is no ultimate medical attention, but currently treatment includes steroids, another form of immunosuppressant, genetically engineered interferon B_{1b} given below the skin, copolymer, or use of another form of inconclusive treatment.

Systemic Diseases

Multiple sclerosis – This is an inflammatory problem of deprivation of the myelin coating in the central nervous system. It results in a number of CNS patches that are scattered in both when they occurred and where they are. Someone who lives in northern latitude has a greater chance of getting it. There is a smaller chance of getting it if another close family member has it. In matched pairs of monozygotic twins, the incidence is 25%. MS may arise at any stage of life, but in general the person will be between 20 and 40, and men are twice as likely to get it. The patient is more often white than black. Neoroophthalmologic elements include afferent or efferent problems, nystagmus, cerebellum problems, saccadic irregularities or cranial nerve disorders in very uncommon instances. When identifying, the attributes are as follows:

- Indication in the neurological system which goes on for longer than 24 hours
- Clinical proof of lesion
- Paraclinical proof of lesion
- Lab results
- Another lesion

Thyroid disease – 20% to 50% of people with hyperthyroid also get thyroid eye disease. This may arise when the person has Hashimoto's thyroiditis, it may arise in every thyroid situation, 20% to 40% demonstrate this condition when a bodily problem is identified, and the majority of people will get it inside of a year and a half of identification of the bodily problem. It is more likely to be found in a female (4:1 to 7:1). Indications may be found in the body, such as agitation, touchiness, lack of physical strength, lessened body weight, sensation of rapid heartbeat, involuntary shaking, perspiration, fast heart rate, shortness of breath, loose bowel movements, lack of tolerance for heat, mood swings, inability to sleep, greater food cravings, enlarged thyroid, thyroid bruit or thrill. In the skin, the patient may experience a disease of the skin, damp skin, pretibial swelling in the skin, loss of pigment in the skin, loss of hair, and brittleness.

Under examination, you may see dysthyroid progressive muscle weakness. Under assessment, look at the thyroid workings in the body, do an imaging study of the orbit, and look for signs of CT. Medical attention includes managing the thyroid, watching, quitting the use of cigarettes, raising head while sleeping, tinted lenses and prednisone (10 days, then quick taper). Other methods include pre-radioactive iodine treatment on a temporary bases, radiation treatment, exposure corneal dystrophy, lid retraction, eye misalignment treatment and orbital decompression treatment. Similar symptoms may indicate arterialized veins in the orbit, uncontrolled cell growth, inferior expansion from paranasal sinuses, severe inflammation of muscle tissue in the orbit, too much growth hormone, severe expansion including cardiac muscle inflammation in the body, trichinosis, and ultrasound of muscles.

Myasthenia gravis – This condition is in the skeletal muscle acetylcholine (Ach) receptors. It creates a problem in the nerve and muscle communications along with a range of frail muscles. It is linked to a tumor in the thymus, thyroid disease, or another form of autoimmune problem. The patient is more likely to be male if it is ocular myasthenia (OM) (57:43), with a mean age of 38;

more likely to be female in generalized myasthenia (GM) (41:59), with a mean age of 33; more likely to be female with female if both conditions are combined together, In any case, the person is generally younger than 40, and the condition may arise in babyhood or as a child. There is no penchant for one ethnicity. With OM, the person may see two images instead of one or droopy lids. With GM, the patient experiences a weak body, such as problems swallowing or problems in the limbs.

Medical attention in the eye includes a patch, ptosis crutch, prism (although this does not generally help since the deviation ranges), drugs such as mestinon and prednisone, operation for strabismus or ptosis, plasmapheresis, removal of the thymus gland, and immunosuppressives. 90% ultimately get indications in the eye. In the beginning, 75% will have droopy lids, but 90% as time goes by. You may see a lid convulsion and ophthalmoparesis. Do a tensilon assessment, neostigmine, anti-ACh receptor antibodies, electromyography and repetitive stimulation assessments in some instances, see a neurologist, and do a chest CT to make sure it is not thymoma.

According to the 1990 Amaurosis Fugax Study Group, the advisable qualities include:

- More than 75% of restricted blood vessel
- Obvious gain in a number of studies
- People with indications are the only ones
- No big danger of having an operation
- Smaller than 2% for perioperative CEA morbidity and mortality rate
- Index attention on a person-by-person basis
- Lack of noteworthy heart or lung problems
- Not obese
- Under 75 years old
- Use of medical attention by itself in 0% to 29% narrowing of blood vessels
- Benefits for 30% to 69% is inconclusive

Carotid Disease

Carotid disease and carotid surgery – Following hemispheric transient ischemic attack (TIA), the danger is 8% each year of getting CVA. Of these, 20% occur inside the beginning month; 50% inside the initial year. 23% have a higher chance in the first 3 years. Following transient visual loss (TVL), the danger is 2% each year, but there is not any quality research for cases that have had no medical attention. Following four-and-a-half years, around 6% get CVA and 11% get tissue death in the retina. In 2 years, the chance of CVA is 17% for TVL and 44% for TIA. Following small clots in the blood of the retina, the chance of CVA is 3% to 5% every year.

North American symptomatic carotid endarterectomy trial – they found that surgical removal of clots in the carotid helped people that had high-grade narrowed blood vessels from 70% to 99%. Research for 30% to 69% of narrowing is not finished.

Transient Visual Loss Indications

Transient visual loss could be in one or both eyes, and could go one for moments, minutes, or hours. This could be a response due to something in the eye, orbit or cranium. The patient may experience a range of sudden onset to slow onset. When it is a gaze loss when viewing a certain side, this indicates a mass in the orbit that either squeezes or elongates as the eye moves around. Look for indications of carotid oxygen deficiency, such as one-sided loss of senses or weakness, problems forming words, temporary loss of sight in one eye, or homonymous hemianopsia in very uncommon instances. Look for indications of migraine, including march (slowly enlarging location of lessened sight) and buildup (worsening of problem within 15 – 20 minutes). Other indications of migraine include head pain, lessened sight the perception of twinkling light around gaps in sight (although lack of this does not rule out migraine). Try to observe the person while the problem is occurring. Look for past migraine problems.

Make sure it is not due to something that results in TVL, and examine the fundus. Rule out problems in the eye, migraine and swelling in the optic nerve. Check for flare-up, blood clots, and thromboembolism. Check for heart problems; look for inflamed blood vessels, and embolism in the heart. Make sure it is not a problem with blood coagulability if the person is young. Think about GCA if the person is elderly. Medical attention includes treatment for the reason the person is having the problem or swollen optic nerve, treatment for migraine or heart disease, managing chances of stroke, use of antiplatelet drug such as aspirin, surgical removal of blood clots when needed, and attention for heart disease.

Trials and Studies

Ischemic optic neuropathy decompression trial – They found that decompression of the optic nerve will not benefit the sight with nonarteritic anterior ION. They found that it might hurt the outcome. Getting better with no medical attention had more benefit in than prior accounts.

Optic neuritis treatment trial – Although they found quicker gaining back of sight when using methylprednisolone into the veins, the ultimate sight in 30 days was comparable in the three groups. In a year, vision was 20/40 or better for 93% of people. There was a higher instance of reappearing optic neuritis with the group that used prednisone taken by mouth, and this was nearly two times more. The use of steroids by mouth or into the vein lessened the instances of clinically definite MS inside the beginning 2 years, but at 3 years, the result was insignificant.

European carotid surgery trial – It helps people with 70% to 99% of narrowing in the carotid. The problems from the operation are worse than the help with 0% to 29% narrowing. For people with 30% to 69% of carotid narrowed vessels, research is unfinished.

Mayo asymptomatic carotid endarterectomy study – Unfinished prior to finding helpful information due to heightened tissue death in the heart muscle mass following holding back the use of aspirin.

Plastic Surgery and Orbital Diseases

Orbit Measurements and Bones

Orbit measurements: volume – 30cc; height – 35mm; width – 40mm; medial wall length – 45mm; globe to optic canal – 18mm; optic nerve – 25mm; intrascleral – 1mm; intraorbital – 25 to 30mm; orbital canal – 10mm; intracranial – 10mm.

Bones in the orbit: sphenoid, ethmoid (which is the thinnest one), zygomatic, maxillary, frontal, lacrimal, palatine.

Dermoid and Epidermoid Cysts

Dermoid and epidermoid cysts is a form of congenital orbital tumor beginning in the early lifespan, this is a smooth cystic mass in the side or above and to the side of the orbit. Use CT scan to recognize the difference between one that is above and toward the midline and encephalocele lesions. If it is dermoid, it is a cyst with an inside layer of keratinized skin and attached parts like hairs and sebaceous glands. If it is epidermoid, the cyst will have an inside layer of keratinized skin but will not have the other attached parts. Medical attention includes cutting it out. If the cyst breaks there will be significant flare-up.

Orbital Cellulitis

An infection in the orbit due to fungus or bacteria can happen in a child or grown person and create peril to the sight and outcome of peril to the person's life. Preseptal celllutitis only happens in the periopbital regions which are in the front of the septum. Orbital cellulitis affects regions towards the back and generally happens along with an active paranasal sinus disease or injury which is linked to an infection in a abrasion of the face. The cause for orbital cellulitis may be in the periorbital region, intraorbital region, from something outside such as injury or an operation, something produced in the brain or body or an organism. To assess, do a culture o Gram stain, CBC, CT, tissue study, fungus, and aspergillus and mucor assessments. This problem may worsen, beginning as preseptal and moving to be orbital cellutitis, then cavernous sinus thrombosis or intracranial abscess if the person does not receive medical attention. When subperiosteal abscesses are created, the person may quickly lose sight.

Antibiotics (contingent upon tests), treatment from otolaryngologist for sinus disease, treatment for mucormycosis if the person is a diabetic or immunosuppressed and has this very unlikely condition, antibiotics by mouth if there is preseptal celllutitis (unless into the vein is needed), another CT scan to look for abscess if there is no improvement in 2 to 4 days, operation to drain abscess, and attention for aspergillosis when needed. Drugs depend on the case. Each person has to be carefully watched. Similar symptoms indicate flare-up in the orbit with no known cause, carotid cavernous fistula or inflamed blood vessels in the orbit.

Thyroid Orbitopathy

Seven Classes Thyroid Orbitopathy:

Class 0 – patient has no indications

Class 1 – just signs, like pulled-back top lid

Class 2 – inflammation in soft tissue periorbital area

Class 3 – abnormal bulging of the eye out of the socket

Class 4 – participation of muscles next to (but not in) eyeball; double vision

Class 5 – participation of cornea; exposure

Class 6 – mild loss due to pressure in optic nerve

Most frequently seen form of proptosis in either one or both eyes for fully-grown people which arises in half of people that have Graves' disease. This condition can be overactive thyroid gland, deficient thyroid gland or a normal thyroid gland. Eye problems which go along with this condition are eye exposure, eye misalignment and pressure on the optic nerve. The patient may experience lid retraction or lag, swelling and fluid in the periorbit, conjunctival chemosis, enlarged vessels over rectus muscle insertions, corneal exposure, ulceration, problems with movement outside the eye, raised IOP, or pressure on the optic nerve. The person is generally from 25 to 50 years old and more likely to be female (8:1). Medical attention includes aids for the local area such as man-made drops, moisturizers, raising the head while sleeping, etc. Corticosteroids may be used. Other options are radiation to the orbit, surgery, decompression on the orbit, surgery on the muscles next to the eye, an operation on the lid margin position, or blepharoplasty. Check the thyroid and do an imaging study of the orbit. In 6 to 18 months, the significant flare-up moves on to be an ongoing, static fibrotic phase. Unprompted getting better and getting worse may happen. Disease in the thyroid and in the orbit are separate from each other, but disease in the orbit can get worse following radioactive iodide thyroid gland management. When a person does not have noteworthy proptosis there still may be abnormal optic nerve functioning because of the pressure. Half of people that have pulled-back top lid will get better with no medical attention. When proptosis gets to its worst state, it will stay the same (but will not get better). The ability to move alters when the acute stage is occurring. Similar symptoms may indicate flare-up in the orbit with no known cause, amyloidosis in the orbit, carotid cavernous fistula, a tumor in the orbit, or a pulled-back eyelid.

Idiopathic Orbital Inflammation

Idiopathic orbital inflammation, also called orbital pseudotumor: significant flare-up with no known cause generally hurts and can be scattered or in one certain place in the orbit. Other conditions should be eliminated prior to identifying the problem as orbital flare-up with no known cause. Medical attention includes looking at scan of the orbit, NSAIDS when there is inflammation in the muscle tissues, prednisone by mouth (for months, with a slow taper), steroids (which usually gives a quick and good result), a tissue study of the orbit in a case which is not getting better or that comes back again, and irradiation or cytoxic agents for people that have cases that are not getting better. Similar symptoms in a fully-grown person may indicate inflamed tissue in the orbit or another problem such as sarcoidosis, Wegener's granulomatosis or Srogen syndrome. In a child, similar symptoms may indicate inflamed tissue in the orbit, break of dermoid cyst, malignant tumor in the muscle tissue, metastatic cancer in the nervous system or leukemic orbital infiltrate.

Indications of this condition include flare-up in the anterior orbit or scattered flare-up. There may be hurting, red lids, fluid and swelling in the lids, swelling in the conjunctiva, lessened sight, lessened movement next to (but outside) the eyeball and general eye inflammation. In an unusual instance there will only be hurting, lessened sight and lessened movement next to (but outside) the eyeball. If there are inflamed muscle tissues, there will be hurting when the eye is moved, lessened ability to move next to (but outside) the eyeball, and chemosis in one place. If there is flare-up in the lacrimal area, there will be hurting, chemosis in one spot, and a lid that is curved like an S. This condition occurs in any stage of life and in both genders. In a child, there may be inflammation in the papilla. To assess, do a CT scan. The consequences of this condition include polymorphous oozing into the flared-up cells such as lymphocytes, neutrophils, plasma cells and macrophages.

Congenital Orbital Tumors

Capillary hemangioma – Beginning in the initial few weeks after birth, this gets bigger in the first year and rolls inward as the years go by. It is a skin-deep strawberry type lesion or a shade of deep blue in the orbit. Kassabach-Merritt syndrome is a prominent aspect and is that is linked to a low platelet count. Manage the lazy eye, eye misalignment or difference in refractive error. Besides this, the case should be watched for rolling inward. Steroids may be used. An operation is only beneficial for deep tumors with good boundaries.

Lymphangioma – Not confined to one area, infiltrative lesion on the lid which begins in the first ten years of life. It quickly gets bigger when it bleeds into the lymphangioma. This is called a chocolate cyst. It gets bigger if an upper respiratory tract infection occurs. Manage the lazy eye, eye misalignment or difference in refractive error. Drain the blood. Since it is infiltrative, an operation is not recommended. When necessary, debulk the lesion in the front.

Cavernous hemangioma – Most frequently seen type of main orbital tumor that is not dangerous to health in fully-grown people, especially females in the middle of the lifespan. There is slowly worsening drooping in the lids, lessened sight due to pressure on the optic nerve and farsightedness as another consequence. It is enclosed and made up of big, enlarged areas that are occupied with red blood cells. Medical attention includes cutting out the lesion in an operation if it puts the eye performance in danger.

Hemangiopericytoma – Not seen very often, a tumor that arises in the middle of the lifespan. It is comparable to cavernous hemangioma and might have a result of fluid in the conjunctiva, displacement, and limitation in the ability to move. Big pericytes are all around the capillaries. Cut it out totally with an operation. It can come back, become malignant or spread to another part of the body.

Neural Tumors

Optic nerve glioma – No hurting, there is bulging of the eyeball out of the socket, lessened sight, and afferent fault in the pupil. The chiasm may be affected. An imaging study will show a bigger than normal optic canal (more than 6.5mm across the center) when plain film is used. You will see a bigger than normal optic nerve that is formed like an S and fusiform with a CT scan. An MRI will give a better assessment when looking at how far back the tumor goes. Medical attention is debatable due to the range of how these tumors get bigger. Some get bigger very quickly, others are slow or do not grow. Watch it, cut it out, or use radiation. Cutting it out includes optic nerve resection with an outcome of blindness. Cut it out in the direction of the chiasm, for corneal exposure or for a proptotic eye with no sight. Radiation is utilized when the tumor cannot be resection and it is going into the chiasm. Optic nerve glioma is made up of cells that look like fibers, a nervous system tumor that includes Rosenthal fibers which arises in the first ten years of life, and 25% to 50% are linked to neurofibromatosis type 1.

Plexiform neurofibromas – Penetrating tumor with many blood vessels inside the lid and orbit (bag of worms), lesion on the top lid, lid that is formed like an S, linked to neurofibromatosis type 1, and greater chance of glaucoma on the same side. It is formed of twisted together bunches of Schwan cells, axons and endoneural fibroblasts. Medical attention includes carefully debunking the lesion.

Rhabdomyosarcoma – Tissue sample study as soon as possible. Do medical tests for metastatic elements in order to find out the stage of the condition. The best treatments are radiation and chemotherapy. These treatments allow 95% of people a 5-year survival rate. Similar symptoms may indicate cellulitis in the orbit, flare-up in the orbit with no known cause, neuroblastoma, lymphangioma including bleeding, capillary hemangioma or broken dermoid cyst.

Meningioma – there are two locations:

1. In the cranium - more frequently seen, occurs in females in the middle of the lifespan, an influence in the sphenoid bone is frequently seen, and there may be bulging of the eye out of the socket, chemosis, swelling and fluid in the lid, temporal fullness and lessened sight as time goes by. Use CT. Cut it out if causing loss of sight, movement or exposure. Use resection and debulking together.
2. In the optic nerve - likely to be in a female in the middle of the lifespan or a kid with neurofibromatosis. There will be an eye that is bulging out of the socket, swelling or wasting away in the optic nerve, optociliary shunt vessels and wrinkles in the choroid. Use CT or MRI. Watch the patient for problems. Use resection if there is a danger of it going into the cranium, gradually worsening or with bad sight. Cut it totally out when there is no sight and the tumor is worsening.

Mesenchymal Tumors

Rhabdomyosarcoma – Most frequently seen form of main malignancy in the eye during the early years (7 to 8 years old). It has to be checked when a child has a quick beginning of a problem in the orbit's function. Study a sample tissue from the lesion when it could be likely. Because of the utilization of chemotherapy and radiation treatments, the percentage of people who continue living following the identification of this condition greatly has gotten better. The patient may experience a quick beginning of proptosis in one eye, flare-up in the lid, injection and bruising. Hurting and lessened sight do not occur very often. Evaluation may show proptosis, down and to the side dislocation of the globe, droopy eyelids, swelling and fluid in the lid and red skin. The patient may have lymph node problems in certain areas of the body which can move out and be metastatic. Do CT, biopsy (right away) and an organized sequence of metastatic tests.

There are four forms, including:

- Embryonal – most frequently seen; located in the orbit's superior nasal quadrant; slack bundles of undifferentiated spindle cells which have no special function and very uncommon crossed grooves.
- Alveolar – worst in terms of malignancy; located in the inferior orbit; containing fibrous and vascular tissue into sections with an inside layer of rhabdomyoblasts.
- Pleomorphic – least commonly seen; arises in fully-grown people; specialized and including effortlessly found crossed grooves.
- Botyroid embryonal – alternative type of embryonal form which arises like bunches of grapes and is penetrated by the paranasal sinuses or conjunctiva.

This condition worsens to become a tumor that includes bony penetration and spreads out into the lymph nodes, lung, bone marrow and brain. The prediction for the future is contingent upon the stage and the elements of how the cells have changed. Grown person pleomorphic has a better prediction than embryonal and botyroid. Embryonal and botyroid have a better prediction than alveolar.

Fibrous histiocytoma – Histiocytic cells in a whorled pattern. The four forms include fibrous dysplasia, ossifying fibroma, osteoma and osteogenic sarcoma. This condition is the most frequently seen form of mesenchymal tumor that is found in the orbit. It occurs in fully-grown people in the middle of the lifespan. The patient may experience bulging of the eyeball out of the socket and lessened sight. It varies and may be benign or malignant. It comes back in the same area. It is very uncommon for it to spread. A CT will show it to have definite boundaries and be of uniform structure. Medical attention includes doing an operation for a totally remove it.

Histiocytosis X – Penetrating granulomatous fixed macrophage. It is a sensitive, obvious mass with rhinorrhea. It occurs due to irregular gatherings of specific histiocytes and Langerhans cells. Elements of this condition include eosinophilic granuloma, Hand-Schüller-Christian syndrome and Letterer-Siwe. Use an electron microscope. Medical attention includes ionizing radiation on the region, cytotoxins and steroids.

Histiocytic Tumors

Lymphocytic tumors -- A histiocytic tumor which is lymphoproliferative, predictably changes from benign to malignant and has the possibility of becoming systemic. It worsens with time, slowly becomes a bulging eye out of the socket, does not hurt, agitates the ability to move, in both eyes for 25% of people and affects the lacrimal gland. It is an orange-pink area in the subconjunctiva. The lumps are not soft and located in the frontal orbit. It arises in the 60s and 70s (very uncommon in childhood). There may be lymphoma in the body. Assess with CT or MRI and do a check of the body. The forms include benign reactive lymphoid hyperplasia, atypical lymphoid hyperplasia and lymphoma. When a person has a lymphoid lesion in the orbit, this condition may arise up to years afterwards. Medical attention includes a tissue sample, ionizing radiation from 1000 – 2500 rads when it is benign reactive or atypical lymphoid hyperplasia, ionizing radiation from 2000 – 4000 rads when it is lymphoma and chemotherapy if it is spreading. Similar symptoms may indicate a lesion in the orbit which has spread, tumor in the lacrimal gland or tumor in the plasma cells.

Lacrimal gland tumors – May be inflammatory, lymphoid or epithelial. Epithelial is the form that makes up half of these tumors, and 50% of these are benign while 50% are malignant adenoma. Use CT. If it is epithelial, the tumor can be benign mixed, malignant mixed or adenoid cystic carcinoma. Medical attention includes getting relevant past medical accounts, making sure it is not an inflammation or infection, imaging assessment, tissue sample study or cutting out the lacrimal gland in total when needed. If it is benign mixed, it has to be totally taken out with no tissue sample first since the orbit could be seeded and the problem could come back or become malignant.

Metastatic Orbital Tumors

Metastatic orbital tumors include:

- Pediatric – comes from neuroblastoma. Elements include the main tumor located in the abdomen, area between the lungs or neck. Spreads into inferior orbit and commonly includes ecchymotic irregular bulging of the eyeball out of the socket.
- Pediatric – comes from leukemia. Acute lymphoblastic leukemia is the most frequently seen. Granulocytic sarcoma can arise prior to indications in the blood or bone marrow.
- Adult – comes from the breast. Most frequently seen type of spreading cancer for females. The woman commonly has had prior breast tissue cancer. It can have an outcome of the eye sinking into the socket, movement problems and droopy lids.
- Adult – comes from the lung. Most frequently seen type of spreading cancer for males. There is not always a prior case of lung carcinoma in the person.

Secondary tumors in the orbit may be in the conjunctiva, globe, lid, sinus or brain.

Orbital Traumas

Midfacial fractures –three Le Fort categorizations:

- Le Fort I – across the lower width maxillary fracture which does not influence the orbit
- Le Fort II – shaped like a pyramid, a fracture that affects the nasal, lacrimal and maxillary bones, middle orbital walls are affected as well
- Le Fort III – skull and face dysjunction; observe to see if the airway is in danger. Affects lateral wall, floor and medial wall.

Orbital wall fractures – Do a CT scan to look for indications. Possible locations:

- Medial wall – operation to fix muscle entrapment or telecanthus. When there are no other indications, watch, instruct the person to refrain from blowing nose; antibiotics may be used when needed
- Roof of the orbit – operation to fix it along with neurosurgery when there are other dislodged fractures
- Zygoma – (tripod fracture) – fix any dislodged or otherwise resulting fractures
- Optic canal – may use high dosage of steroids into the vein when needed; decompression including an operation for evacuating the nerve sheath hematoma is debatable

Orbital floor fracture – This is an injury to the floor of the orbit and is a blowout fracture when the rim is unaffected. A blowout is most frequently found on the posteromedial region of the orbital floor. It can have an outcome of eye sinking into the socket and double vision. The problem is generally fixed one to two weeks following the problem when there is sinking of the eye into the socket, double vision that affects a purposeful gaze or big fracture. Noncircuitous force on the rim creates a fracture, pressure force on the rim creates buckling and has an outcome of a floor fracture and greater amounts of pressure in the orbit can result in a slender part of the floor becoming fractured. In the beginning the patient may experience swelling and fluid in the lid, bruising, a bulging eye or an eye that sinks in. The patient may have double vision and suborbital decreasing of nerve sensitivity. Make sure it is not nerve disorder due to injury. Use plain film and CT. Watch progression for a week to see if it gets better of affects movement. Ongoing problems with movement may be due to entrapment, muscles outside (but near) the eye or nerve harm. When a big fracture is not fixed, an outcome of a sunken in eye may occur as time goes by. Use ice packs, antibiotics if needed, and refrain from blowing the nose. Surgery will be needed in one to two weeks when there is entrapment, sinking that is more than 2mm or a fracture that affects half (or more) of the floor.

Orbital emphysema – May result in greater pressure in the orbit and artery block. It sometimes can be examined by feeling the air under the skin. When the sight is not harmed, watch the patient's case. When sight is affected or if there is an artery block, put a needle into the air pocket and draw it off it into a syringe that is full of water.

Orbital foreign bodies – X-ray or CT to find the region, but do not use MRI if the element is made of metal. Take it out when it is made of vegetable matter or when it is in the front and has sharp borders. Just watch the case when it is in the back of if it is not affecting the person.

Later complications of anophthalmic socket – It may be that the volume in the orbit is lacking including deep superior depression, slackness or turning out of the bottom lid and droopy lids. Change out the spherical implant in the orbit for one with bigger dimensions or utilize a flat subperiosteal orbital implant on the floor of the orbit. It may be that the socket is reduced in size, including inability to keep prosthesis and lack of or inadequate fornices. Medical attention choices include buccal mucus membrane graft, hard palate graft to reshape the fornix to go along with lateral plastic surgery on the canthus and dermis fat graft.

Orbital hemorrhage – Top and bottom lid bruising and bleeding in the conjunctiva with lessened ability for the eye to move, a chance of greater tension in the orbit, lessened ability to see, afferent fault in the pupil, heightened IOP and central artery block in the retina. When it occurs following an operation, undo the incision and get the clot out. When it may put the sight in danger, do lateral surgical division of the canthus and break down of inferior limb of lateral canthal tendon. For a lessened IOP use mannitol, acetazolamide, timolol or apraclonidine. When the pressure in the orbit and globe is raised and stays that way and there is a block or throbbing in the central artery in the retina, decompression may be used.

Eyelid Structure

Müller's Muscle

- Supplied by a sympathetic nerve
- Begins in the bottom surface of levator muscle close to where the levator muscle changes to be aponeurosis.
- Goes into superior border of tarsus.

Orbicularis Muscle

- Opening/closing muscle helps lids shut; element of lacrimal pump.
- Supplied by cranial nerve VII.
- Split into pretarsal, preseptal and orbital
- Pretarsal and preseptal are unthinking, like blinking, but orbital works for purposeful shutting, like wink or blepharospam.
- Pretarsal segments in lids include medial add-on in front; element of front limb in medial canthal tendon, medial add-on in back, Horner's tensor tarsi muscle; goes in back of canaliculi to connect to lacrimal crest in back. The top and bottom lid pretarsal orbicularis muscles come together in lateral canthal region to be element of lateral canthal tendon.
- Preseptal segments in lids include medial attachment in front. This turns into element of anterior limb in medial canthal tendon, medial posterior attachment, Jones' muscle, enters lacrimal diaphragm of tear sac. To the side, preseptal muscles create lateral palpebral raphe that goes on top of lateral rim of orbit.
- Orbital segment comes from front limb of medial canthal tendon and periosteum. It goes around the orbit.

Orbital Septum

- Wall in the middle of the lid and the rest of the orbit that restricts disbursement of infection or bleeding; in back of orbicularis muscle and in front of orbital fat.
- Slender sheet of fiber comes up from periosteum on top of superior and inferior rims of the orbit, and then goes into the middle of the posterior lacrimal crest and to the side slightly in front of the side tubercle in the orbit.
- In the top lid, septum joins together with the levator aponeeurosis about 4mm on top of the superior tarsal border if the person is white, but the measurement is nearer if the person is Asian.
- In the low lid, septum joins together with capsulopalpebral fascia around 4mm underneath the inferior tarsal edges for a white person. The whole thing, together with the inferior tarsal smooth muscle, goes into the tarsus.

Eyelid Fat Pads

- Found in back of the orbital septum for top and bottom lids.
- Top lid – two preaponeurotic fat pads; medial is whiter; displaced lacrimal gland in the orbit is sometimes misidentified as a side fat pad.
- Bottom lid – three fat pads; the inferior oblique muscle goes in the middle of the medial and central fat pads.

Capsulopalpebral Fascia

- Comes up from inferior rectus muscle, splits and goes around inferior oblique muscle
- In front of the inferior oblique muscle the two sections connect to create Lockwood's suspensory ligament.
- Goes more into the anterior, propels strands into inferior conjunctival fornix on top of orbicularis muscle and skin.
- Goes into inferior tarsus

Inferior Tarsal Muscle

- Supplied by sympathetic nerve (like Müller's muscle).
- Initiates on back surface of capsulopalpebral fascia.
- Goes into inferior edge of tarsus including capsulopalpebral fascia.

Levator Palpebrae Superioris Muscle

- Lifts top lid
- Supplied by cranial nerve III.
- Begins on apex of orbit on top of annulus of Zinn; ~40mm in length.
- Whitnall's ligament is short version of anterior sheath in levator muscle. It works like a lever around which aponeurosis in superior orbit turns. It connects in the middle to tissue around trochlea and superior oblique tendon. In the side, it propels septae through stroma and curves up to connect to inside of lateral orbital wall; ~10mm on top of lateral orbital tubercle.
- It turns aponeurosis around 14 – 20mm on top of superior tarsal edge; middle horn of aponeurosis goes into posterior lacrimal crest; side horn splits orbit and palpebral lobes of lacrimal gland and goes into side orbital tubercle.
- Aponeurosis splits to be anterior and posterior segments 3-4mm on top of superior border of tarsus; frontal part propels fibers to orbicularis and skin on top to create crease in top lid. Back part goes into front surface of bottom 2/3 of tarsus.

Tarsus

- Unyielding, thick connective tissue that is not cartilage.
- Top lid plate is 9-10mm from top to bottom.
- Bottom lid plate is 4mm or smaller from top to bottom.
- It is 1mm in thickness and tapers medially and laterally.

Palpebral Conjunctiva

- Layer of lids farthest to the back.
- Inside, there are accessory lacrimal glands of Krause and Wolfring. These are in charge of basal tear secretion and goblet cells that make mucus.

Medial canthal tendon – The superior and inferior limbs of it come up from medial elements of tarsal plates and orbicularis muscle, divide in the front and back and wrap around the lacrimal sac. They go into the front and back lacrimal crests.

Lateral Canthal Tendon:

- Superior and inferior limbs come up from the side elements of tarsal plates and orbicularis muscle. They go into the inside of the lateral rim of the orbit on the side tubercle of the orbit.
- Goes in 3mm above the medial canthal tendon.

Lateral orbital tubercle, or Whitnall's –Connected to it are the side canthal tendon, side retinaculum and Lockwood's ligament. Look at ligament of lateral rectus muscle and side horn of levator aponeurosis.

Eyelid margin – Includes, in order of front to back, the eyelash follicles, muscle of Riolan, meibomian gland orifices and conjunctiva.

Vascular Supply for the Lids

- Inside carotid by means of the eye's support and the branches that come from it which are above the eye and in the tears.
- Outside carotid by means of arteries in the face which are angular and toward the temple.
- In the top lid, the marginal arterial support is located 2mm above the edge and in front of the tarsal plate. Peripheral arterial support is located above the tarsus and between aponeurosis and Müller's muscle.
- In the low lid, there is commonly a single arterial support on the edge of the inferior tarsal.

Venous Drainage

- Pretarsal tissues are drawn off to angular vein in the middle an to the superficial temporal vein on the side.
- Posttarsal tissues are drawn off to veins in the orbit and the far branches of the frontal vein in the face and the pterygoid plexus.

Sensory Nerve Supply:

- Branches of the eye's portion of trigeminal nerve, which is V_1, supplies the forehead, top lid, side and middle periocular regions and tip of nose.
- Branches of the maxillary portion, which is V_2, supplies the bottom lid and area in the cheek.

Standard Lid Dimensions:

- Margin reflex distance 1 (MRD_1) – 4mm, beginning from the top lid margin and going to the pupillary light reflex
- Margin reflex distance 2 (MRD_2) – 6mm, beginning from the bottom lid margin and going to the pupillary light reflex
- Palpebral fissure height – 10mm, from the top lid to the bottom lid
- Upper lid crease height – ranges, contingent upon male/female; Caucasian male is 9-10mm, female is 8-9mm; Asian is 1-10mm and 12-15mm
- Levator muscle function (LF) – 12-15mm, journey of the top lid beginning in downgaze and going to upgaze with a stationary brow so that the frontalis muscle does not move

Ectropion

Ectropion is when the margin of the lid turns out. The patient may experience aggravation in the eye, red eye, tears, and a slack bottom lid which falls out from the globe. You may see horizontal slackness in the lid and scarring on the skin, increased size of the papillary on the bare eyelid membrane and a chance of keratinization, gathered tears on the bottom lid and inferior exposure keratopathy. As time goes by, a turned out lid margin could have an outcome of keratinization in the conjunctiva and punctual scars. A person with exposure keratopathy may also get an infection in the cornea. Punctual ectropion and a slack lid could cause a problem of a watery eye.

Ectropion forms and medical attention:

- Present at birth – No medical attention needed except moisturizing with manmade tears or cream; when significant or if it has indications, the anterior lamella has to be elongated vertically utilizing a skin graft
- Involutional – Slackness across is treated with a tightening process such as lateral canthoplasty; another option is to try reinsertion on the bottom lid retractors
- Paralytic - Just watch the case when transitory; when it is enduring, use horizontal tightening
- Cicatricial – Steroid massage or injection for half of a year in a significant case. When that is finished, an operation may be done; scar bands may be destroyed as long as the lid is on stretch; lacking skin can be fixed with lateral canthoplasty and total-thickness skin graft
- Inflammatory – Anything causing a reaction should be stopped; utilize steroid balm or injection for swelling; operation is done just like in a cicatricial case
- Mechanical – Cut out tumors; when it also has cicatricial elements, do a total-thickness skin graft

Ectropion Causes:

- Present at birth – up-and-down dimensions of frontal lamella; very uncommon; at times is linked to blepharophimosis syndrome
- Involutional – bottom lid slackness, result of growing old and gravity
- Paralytic – paralysis in the face and lessened orbicularis muscle quality in the bottom lid
- Cicatricial – lessening in length of frontal lamella due to heat burn, chemical burn, actinic skin harm, scars from an injury or an operation on the bottom lid
- Inflammatory – lessening in length of frontal lamella due to ongoing flare-up and scars due to rosacea dermatitis, wasting away dermatitis, eczematoid dermatitis, herpes zoster infection or an allergy to ongoing utilization of drops used in the eye
- Mechanical – hulking tumors in the lid

Entropion

Entropion is when the lid margin is turned in; aggravation and red eyes, teary eyes and lid that is turned in to globe. You may see a lid margin and lashes that have curved in and slackness in the lid. If the person has a discontinuous case, it may be drawn out if you ask the person to vigorously press his lids shut. Lashes may be growing inward including inferior bulbar conjunctival injection and conjuncntival swelling and inferior corneal dystrophy. There is potential for cicatricial disease in conjunctiva including trachoma or cicatricial pemphigoid in the eye. As long as the lashes are making contact with the cornea, there will be ongoing collapse of epithelium and chance of scarring, reduction of thickness, puncturing and infection. Similar symptoms may indicate more primary issue due to flare-up, previous operation or tumor, or abnormal eyelash growth. Involutional entropion may be caused by bottom lid slackness, wasting away of orbital fat, preseptal orbicularis oculi muscle superseding the pretarsal orbicularis oculi muscle, or a problem with bottom lid retractors.

Entropion Forms and Medical Attention:

- Present at birth – When slight, fix with a surgical removal of skin and muscle under the margin; when significant, use posterior lamella elongation when needed
- Acute spastic – Manage aggravation with moisturizer; with flare-up inside the eye, use a steroid applied to the area; think about doing Quickert-Rathbun rotation sutures for a short-term basis
- Involutional – Do horizontal tightening, use rotation sutures, total-thickness horizontal blepharotomy cuts and reattachment of bottom lid retractors. These may be done individually or a mixture of them can help achieve a more lasting solution
- Cicatricial – Manage the reason for the problem, stop using anything that could be aggravating the problem, elongate the posterior lamella utilizing a graft along with rotation sutures and plastic surgery of the side canthus

The types of ptosis (droopy eyelids) are as follows: present at birth, myogenic (obtained during life), aponeurotic, neurogenic, mechanical and traumatic.

Entropion causes:

- Present at birth – Linked to bottom lid retractor faulty development; formation problems on tarsal plate and comparatively undersized length of posterior lamella
- Acute spastic – Eye aggravation or flare-up following eye operation
- Involutional – Mixture of slackness across bottom lid, weakening or tearing in bottom lid retractors and domination of preseptal over pretarsal orbicularis muscle
- Cicatricial – Undersized length in posterior lamella by cicatricial procedures in the conjunctiva; OCP, Steven-Johnson syndrome, trachoma, herpes zoster, enucleation, heat burn, chemical burn, ongoing utilization of drops in the eyes.

Eyelid Faults

Ankyloblepharon – Joined together lids incompletely or totally with skin webs.

Blepharophimosis syndrome – Inherited autosomal dominant; marked with these three things: wide-set eye opening, epicanthus inversus and droopy lids.

Coloboma – Cleft is generally in the middle of the top lid, can be linked to another form of cleft in the face, lacrimal malformation and Goldenhar syndrome; try not to utilize lid-sharing processes such as Hughes and Cutler-Beard for fixing it in a baby or child since this can result in occlusion amblyopia.

Distichiasis – Present at birth or obtained later; another row of lashes that go by the place where the meibomian glands open; in the beginning, use moisturizers and soft contacts. Operation options include cold therapy, lid splitting including cold therapy and cutting out the involved tarsal plate utilizing mucosal graft

Epicanthus – Skin fold in middle of the canthus; forms include tarsalis, where it stands out the most on the top lid, inversus, where fold stands out the most in the bottom lid, and palpebralis, where fold is evenly allocated

Epiblepharon – Extra pretarsal orbicularis muscle and skin take precedence over the lid margin and work to make the lashes go up or in to the globe; margin does not become turned in; gets better as time goes by for a lot of kids; an operation might become needed in which a skin strip and orbicularis is cut out under or over the margin so that the fault is shut.

Euryblepharon – Enlarged palpebral fissure is due to elongation of the bottom lid towards the temple and up-and-down diminishing in length; side tendon in the canthus is common dislodged to the inferior; operation utilizes total-thickness block resection on the lid that is affected, moving the side tendon in the canthus back into place and total-thickness skin graft if there is diminished length.

Eyelid retraction – Top and bottom eyelid retraction happens if the MRD_1 is bigger than 4mm and MRD_2 is bigger than 6mm. It is commonly linked to scleral show because that condition can result in eye exposure and aggravation. Retraction is frequently caused by thyroid disease in the eye. It can be present at birth, neurological, contralateral (as with Herring's phenomenon), following surgery, following an injury, or after a vertical muscle operation. Look at how the thyroid is working. The patient may have ongoing problems shutting the lid, particularly involving Bell's reflex. This may cause exposure inflammation in the cornea and has the potential to create holes or infection in the cornea. You may see aggravation and tears, withdrawal of the top lid from where it usually is 2mm under superior limbus, withdrawal of bottom lid from where it usually is on the inferior limbus, an eye that cannot shut all the way, conjunctival injection and corneal dystrophy.

On the top lid, a slight case just needs moisturizing in the eye. It is a medium to bad case, make an indentation in the levator aponeurosis by itself or together with cutting out or making an indentation in Müller's muscle. A spacer graft in the sclera can also be used. In the bottom lid, a slight case just needs moisturizing in the eye. A medium to bad case calls for making an indentation of retractors including grafting and lateral tarsal strip process which are done together.

The benign lesions found on the lids include chalazion, papilloma, verruca vulgaris, seborrheic keratosis, actinic keratosis, keratoacanthoma, molluscum contagiosum, nevus, xanthelasma, juvenile xanthogranuloma, syringoma, trichoepithelioma, hydrocystoma, epithelial inclusion cyst and amyloid.

The malignant tumors found on the lids include basal cell carcinoma (most frequently seen), squamous cell carcinoma, sebaceous cell carcinoma and melanoma.

Tumors on the lids – It is fundamental to identify any potential malignancy. Find out how long the lesion has been there, how it has altered in dimension or in the way it looks, if it is a reappearance of something that has been handled in the past, whether there was past skin cancer and how much sun the person gets. Whenever there is potential for malignancy, do a tissue sample study. Ongoing blepharoconjunctivitis which does not do well with medical attention could be sebaceous carcinoma, so do a biopsy. Since malignant and benign lesions can look alike, go ahead with a biopsy when there is a possibility of it (particularly when the person is aged).

Eyelid Fault Operations

Lateral canthus – Use periosteal flap turned so that it works to be the lateral canthus

Medial canthus – Main healing; total-thickness skin graft; forehead/glabellar flabs may be turned to plug the fault; check lacrimal elements (silicone nasolacrimal intubation could be needed).

Top lid – Small fault involves a quarter or less of the lid margin. Use noncircuitous closure which may include the necessity of getting out the superior crus of the side tendon of the canthus.

Medium fault affects a quarter to half of the margin. Use advance lateral segment on the lid including getting out the superior crus of the side tendon of the canthus by itself or together with semicircular skin flap. A big fault affects half or more of the margin. Use Cutler-Beard.

Bottom lid – Small fault needs noncircuitous closure which may include the necessity of getting out the superior crus of the side tendon of the canthus. Medium needs activation of the side tissue in the lid including getting out the superior crus of the side tendon of the canthus by itself or together with semicircular skin flap. Big needs Hughes tarsoconjunctival flap beginning at the middle of the top lid or from the side top lid including total-thickness skin graft on top or skin advancement flap.

Benign Essential Blepharospasm

Benign essential blepharospasm has an issue in both eyes and is marked with uncontrolled tremors from the orbicularis oculi muscle. The finest medical attention includes botulinum toxin injections. It could be due to heightened excitatory drive because of basal ganglia. The patient's tremors may cause the inability to see. It does not occur when asleep. It is also linked to dryness in the eyes, levator dehiscence ptosis and dermatochalasis. The patient is likely to be a female in her 40's or 50's. You will find that muscle power is regular but there is lessened basal tear emission. This condition begins as slight shuddering and can move on to be powerful muscle contractions which restrict functional sight. Most people are helped with botulinum toxin injections for 3-6 months, but people who are not helped by it may need myectomy operation. Neurectomy is another choice, but it is not used as often since there are inbuilt dangers to it. Dryness can be treated with moisturizers/man-made tears.

Similar symptoms in both eyes may indicate meige syndrome, reflex tremor, a neurodegenerative problem or a condition caused by a drug. It could be hemifacial tremor in one eye. Similar symptoms may indicate distal nerve aggravating lesion in the face, post-facial palsy syndrome, facial myokymia or superior limbic keratoconjunctivitis.

Facial Palsy

Facial palsy - medical attention includes managing it for the time being if the problem is projected to get better. These include moisturizers in the eye, moisture chambers and adhesive tape to close the lids while asleep, something heavy stuck to the lids and short-term tarsorrhaphy. In a case that will not go away, an operation to put a gold weight or palpebral spring on the top lid may be used. Plastic surgery on the side canthus to fix paralytic ectropion may be done. Someone with a new identification of this condition has to be watched very carefully.

Facial palsy can cause failure of the lids to totally close and bare cornea. This has to be managed assertively so that other problems will not arise as well. It may be caused by tumor, injury, infection, operation, inadequate oxygen flow or Bell's palsy with no known cause. The person may not be able to shut the lids, have aggravation, hurting and tears, and the face may be unbalanced with drool and a hard time talking. You may find a pulled back top lid, no movement in the bottom lid ectropion, gathered tears in the bottom cul de sac due to inadequate lacrimal pump, ptosis in the forehead and brow along with dermatochalasis, and Bell's phenomenon. Check for another form of cranial nerve affectation. Suggest that the patient see an atlaryngologist. An MRI may be done, particularly if there is also obtained loss of hearing. In a case where the facial nerve role goes back to normal, watch for peculiar renewal and spasticity in muscles that affect the person's expression.

Eyelid Trauma

Check the patient background and find out if there has been dull or piercing injury, what kind of harm was done and whether the person was unconscious. Check sight in each eye, globe (to make sure there was no rupture), eyelids, orbit and whether the lacrimal system was affected. Search and wash out the lacrimal area to check patency and do CT of the axis of the orbit and the cornea to make sure nothing is broken.

When the lid has a laceration, wash out the area using sterile saline and check for debris. In a case where fat from the orbit has gotten displaced, the septum in the orbit is compromised. Check how the levator is working and fix when it has been torn or cut. Utilize interrupted sutures on the area. Deeper hidden sutures are only utilized when needed.

Only attend to lesser alterations following 6 months. Medical attention in the meantime may include steroid cream massage or steroids put into the lesion.

Lessened tissue – Eyelid has blood vessels, it may be put back even if time has passed. Tissue in the lid ought not to be cut out when the main thing is being fixed.

Margin of the lid is lacerated – Get a quality estimate and turning out of the laceration to have a quality aesthetic and serviceable outcome. Use 6-0 suture (silk) in the gray line on the cut or torn borders of the margin. Do not tie it. That will aid in getting the lid back into place when you are putting in tarsal sutures. Reanastamose the tarsus using two on the bottom eyelid or three on the top eyelid 5-0 absorbable interrupted sutures that do not go all the way through the thickness. Tie the gray-line silk suture but let the ends stay long. Put 6-0 silk suture into the lash line and let the ends stay long. Fix the laceration and use the long ends of the margin sutures with the skin sutures that are nearest.

Medial canthal area – When the medial canthal area is lacerated, search the area, particularly in an instance where the opening is medial to the punctum. When just one canaliculus was harmed use monocanalicular/bicanalicular stent. When they are both affected, use bicanalicular intubation including silicone tubing, then let the stents stay there for a quarter to half of a year. Utilize interrupted 8-0 absorbable sutures for estimating the lacerated borders. Use bigger absorbable sutures for the muscle around it and to shut the skin. Sudden tearing away of surface and deeper heads of the tendon in this area will have an outcome of an increased distance between the inside corners of the eyes. If this happens, you may fix it with a choice of transnasal wiring or fixation screws in the back lacrimal crest.

Burns – A burn is attended with eye and lid moisturizer salve. Use moisture chambers for a temporary amount of time. Later alterations that result from a burn may be handled with skin graft or some form of flap.

LACRIMAL SYSTEM

THE LACRIMAL SYSTEM IS MADE UP OF:

- Canaliculi – 2mm up-and-down, 8mm across, 90% of the top and bottom of it connect to create one canaliculus
- Valve of Rosenmueller – located between the joined-together canaliculus and lacrimal sac, and stops the backflow of tears from the sac into the canaliculus
- Lacrimal sac – 10mm in length, located between front and back crus of the middle tendon in the canthus; back head of preseptal orbicularis muscle goes into the sac
- Nasolacrimal duct – 12mm in length, moves towards the inferoposterolateral area and is done under the inferior turbinate which is 30mm away from external areas in a fully-grown person (20mm in a child).
- Valve of Hasner – mucosal fold located on the distal end of nasolacrimal duct; accountable for nasolacrimal duct blockage which is present at birth

- Lacrimal outflow problems which are present at birth – faulty formation of puntal or canalicular area, hernial protrusion of the lacrimal sac which was present at birth, block in nasolacrimal duct which was present at birth.

Lacrimal pump – tears begin at the punctum into lacrimal sac, lids shut, surface and deep heads of pretarsal orbicularis contract squeeze, ampulla constricts, punctum moves towards the middle, canaliculus becomes smaller across, surface and deep heads of preseptal orbicularis constrict, lacrimal sac draws out and gets bigger to make negative pressure, tears come out from canaliculi into the sac. With lids open, tears go from sac to nose, lacrimal sac gives way and pushes them into the nose, puncta goes to the side and tears go into the canaliculi.

Tearing – Investigate area and wash out, utilize dye disappearance assessment to find any block in flow, Jones 1 primary dye to find a block in structure or utility, Jones 2 secondary dye to find obstacle or problem with pump, CT to find tumors or sinus disease, tear break-up time, basal tear secretion, Schirmer 1 to find a lack in basal and reflex, Schirmer 2 to see lack in reflex tear factor, and dacryocystogram/dacryoscintography to look for an obstacle in structure or purpose. Check for excessive secretion due to reflex tearing which is linked to basal tear lack, disease in the cornea, flare-up or abnormal growth in the lacrimal gland, CNS disease, slit-lamp assessment, fluorescein and rose Bengal staining and tear assessment. Check the placement of the bottom lid including slackness and seventh-nerve utility. Check for a punctual problem including stenosis, blocking or ectropion. Investigate the canaliculus to make sure there is no block. Wash out the nasolacrimal system and check for a block. If the wash goes through, use Jones' assessments to check for an obstruction on a following check-up. If there may be a tumor, do CT.

Lacrimal outflow problems which are obtained following birth – Punctual problems such as narrowed blood vessels, block or abnormal turning out of the lid; canalicular problem such as inflamed tear duct, scars or blocking; lacrimal sac problems such as inflammation in the nasolacrimal sac, mass of minerals in lacrimal sac or duct, tumor; nasolacrimal duct problems such as primary or secondary obtained block.

Medical attention for congenital problems:

- Faulty formation of punctal or canalicular area – An incision down on top of the created ampulla including a lack of an opening could show clearly revealed canaliculus.
- Hernial protrusion of the lacrimal sac – Make sure it is not medial hernia of the brain, attention includes antibiotics applied to the area and massage. When this does not work or if an infection forms, investigate the area.
- Block in nasolacrimal duct – Start with antibiotics on the area and massage, investigate including likelihood of infracture in inferior turbinate once half a year has passed (but prior to 13 months having passed since the investigation will not be as good after that). When ongoing investigations do not help, put in silicone tubes.
- Punctual problems – For narrowed blood vessels or block, do one snip punctoplasty or there is potential for putting in silicone tube. For outward turned eyelid, use medial diamond-wedge resection in the conjunctiva to turn it in or use another form of fixing the problem

Medical attention for obtained problems:

- Canalicular problems – inflammation of the tear duct is treated with warm pads, enlarging and scraping, washing using penicillin, penicillin drops applied to the area and sometimes canaliculotomy including scraping. An incomplete obstruction is treated with putting in a silicone tube stent. Total block is treated with DCR including Jones pyrex tube put in to go around canaliculi.
- Lacrimal sac problems – in an acute case, do not wash out. Use warm pads, antibiotics on the area or in the body, i.v. antibiotics when there is significant infection, cut and drain when the pyocele is pointing, culture assessments, DCR after infection is gone. An ongoing case is treated with DCR. Mass of minerals in lacrimal sac is treated with DCR. Tumor requires CT scan, removal with an operation, irradiation in the case of lymphoid growth
- Nasolacrimal duct problems – Use DCR for both primary and secondary obtained blocks.

Pediatric Ophthalmology

Lid Coloboma

In lid colobomaocal there is a lack in the margin and eyelid which is generally located on the top lid. It may arise by itself or may be linked to another issue like Goldenhar syndrome. It is an irregularity that forms during development. In the eye, there will be a focal lid notch (on the top most of the time), lack of tarsus, eyelashes and meibomian glands, and a bare cornea when the fault is big. Medical attention includes an operation. Steer clear of a lid-sharing process since that may have an outcome of blocking lazy eye. In the body, Goldenhar's syndrome includes coloboma in one or two eyes, skin tags in front of the ear, irregularities in the vertebrae, dermoid in the limbus, abnormally small outer ear and exceedingly wide mouth.

Lid malpositions that are present at birth –Entropion, epiblepharon, epicanthal folds, blepharophimosis and ankyloblepharon.

Ptosis

Causes for ptosis obtained after birth – Horner syndrome, myasthenia gravis, ongoing progressive external ophthalmoplegia, cranial nerve III palsy and Garcus-Gunn synkinesis.

Congenital ptosis – One or both eyes with droopy lids, including restriction in the top lid movement due to the fibrotic levator. The cause is unknown. You may see droopy lids in the main pose, small or lack of levator operation, bad ability to move when downgaze pose is in play and person utilizing the brow to lift the lids. Medical attention includes handling lazy eye when it is an issue, postponing the droopy lid attention when the problem is not blocking the visual axis, and frontalis suspension.

Distichiasis – An extra line of thin eyelashes develops. It is by the meibomian gland openings in many cases. It is seen in kids with Milroy syndrome. These extra lashes are not generally aggravating to the cornea. When the eye is unharmed, no medical attention is needed. Otherwise, medical attention includes a lid-splitting process to take out the back lamella including the irregular lashes.

Trichiasis

Trichiasis is when more lashes go in the wrong direction, generally due to scars on the conjunctiva and a deformed lid margin. This occurs from a number of causes, but generally is it from an infection like trachoma, EKC or another issue like cicatrical pemphigoid in the eye. You may see lashes that go in toward the eye and make contact with the cornea, thick, added lashes in rows, staining in the epithelium, aggravation, and scars on the conjunctiva and lid. Medical attention includes electrolysis or cold therapy on the lash follicles or lid-splitting to take out the added lashes.

Ophthalmia Neonatorum

Ophthalmia neonatorum involves conjunctivitis with pus which arises in the initial month of the lifespan. It is critical to identify the issue and give medical attention to the baby right away. This condition is obtained in the birth canal or perinatal period. There is and pus together to hyperpurulent emission and an affected cornea with gonococcus. There may be extra blood in the conjunctiva and swelling and fluid in the lid.

Infectious and Allergic Disorders

Ophthalmia neonatorum – Linked to Chlamydia in the initial 6 weeks. Medical attention includes Gram stain of the emission with blood, chocolate and Thayer-Martin media. Culture/sensitivity assessments are needed. Gonococcus is handled with third-generation cephalosporins in the body, antibiotics on the skin and saline wash every hour. Serologic assessments for syphilis and HIV are needed when the baby has either gonococcal or Chlamydia. Chlamydia is handled utilizing sulfacetamide 10% salve four times every day for 3 weeks. This will keep pneumonitis from arising. The baby's parents and any other partners should also receive medical attention for Chlamydia or other STDs. Bacterial conjunctivitis has the medical attention of sulfacetamide 10% salve or Polysporin ophthalmic salve three times every day. Treatment to prevent this condition is required in every state with erythromycin salve, tetracycline salve or 1% silver nitrate. A case of toxic conjunctivitis will heal on its own in a few days.

Dacryocystitis - Bacterial infection in the area where liquid flows out of the lacrimal system. It is frequently linked to dacryostenosis which is present at birth. The patient may experience redness in the skin, hurting in the nasal canthal area, and the problem can worsen to become preseptal and eye cellulitis. Medical attention includes antibiotics in the body including Gram-positive coverage. Investigate the lacrimal area after the infection gets better to get out blocks.

Preseptal and orbital cellulitis - The preseptal condition is bacterial infection in the periocular tissues in front of the septum of the eye. It is caused by injury or an infection that came from the paranasal sinus area linked to an upper respiratory tract infection. The patient may experience swelling and fluid in the lid, erythema and vesicular lesions in impetigo. Herpes simplex is sometimes mistaken for impetigo. Medical attention includes antibiotics in the body first, then antibiotics by mouth.

Preseptal and orbital cellulitis - In any case, H. influenzae may be a cause and Staphylococcus and Streptococcus are frequently seen causes after an injury. Similar symptoms may indicate rhabdomyosarcoma, pseudotumor that has flare-up or cavernous sinus thrombosis.

Orbital condition - Infection in the orbit that affects the tissues in back of the septum. It is caused by infiltrating injury in the orbit or ethmoid sinusitis. The patient may experience a bulging eyeball out of the socket, restriction in the eye's movement and afferent fault in the pupil if pressure is on the optic nerve. The following indications are more often orbital, but may be in preseptal: sluggishness, high body temperature, unusually high number of leukocytes and an inflammation in the sinuses. Go to the hospital because the problem may be deadly or impair sight. The person will need antibiotics in the body, CT on the orbit, an otorhinologic appointment to take the fluid out of the access, and mucormycosis may be used when the person has diabetes or is immunosuppressed.

Vernal conjunctivitis - Allergy related conjunctivitis that is marked with getting worse and better depending upon the time of year. It is more frequently seen in male children and in people with prior asthma, hypersensitivity to allergens or eczema. It is caused by pollen or mold particular immunoglobulnies E and G. The patient may experience scratchiness, red eyes and watery emission. You may see swelling and fluid in the lids and conjunctiva, soft and watery swelling and fluid in the conjunctiva, conjunctivitis in the papilla that can result in giant papillae, in the limbus it is marked with nodes of flare-up and white middles, and vernal plaque in the cornea could result in scars on the subepithelial area. Medical attention includes mast cell stabilizers, antihistamine applied to the area, drugs to relieve congestion, man-made tears, allergy aids for the body and steroids on the area (but let the person know about the danger of glaucoma).

Nasolacrimal duct obstruction - Present at birth block of the nasolacrimal duct happens with impotency in the area and is generally because of no perforation on the distal end of the duct the way it is beneath the inferior turbinate. Blocks are frequently seen with craniofacial problems. The patient may experience watery eyes and reflux with mucus when the lacrimal sac presses together.

It is seen in 10% of every baby born. 90% of instances get better with no medical attention by the time the child has a first birthday. Medical attention includes massage on the nasolacrimal sac, antibiotics on the skin and investigation of the duct by the first birthday when the case does not appear to be getting better on its own. Similar symptoms may indicate glaucoma that is present at birth.

Irregularities in the cornea and eye, present at birth – Clerocornea, megalocornea, microcornea, cornea plana, keratoglobus, buphthalmos, nanophthalmos and microphthalmos.

Developmental lacrimal anomalies – Present at birth, not perforated punctum could affect the top and bottom puncta. Present at birth fistulas in the lacrimal sac show up under the middle of the canthus and could arise with another form of developmental irregularity. The patient may experience watering in the eye with a lack of sticky mucus coming out. When the person has canaliculi and no perforation in the punctum, use 25-gauge needle or Bard-Parker #11 blade. With no canaliculi, the person could have to have conjunctivodacryocystorhinostomy.

Dacryocele – Proximal and distal areas are blocked in the lacrimal system; causes bloating/swelling of mucous in the lacrimal sac. The patient may experience a mass in the nasal canthus (inferior to tendon) that is a shade of blue. The person may get an infection as a lesser problem. Use massage and help for the infection. Linked cysts in the nasopharynx can cause a problem in respiration. Investigation in the beginning of the lifespan can give healing properties. Similar symptoms may indicate encephalocele, meningomyelocele or hemangioma.

Dysgenesis and Opacities

Anterior segment dysgenesis – Also called mesodermal dysgenesis and anterior chamber cleavage syndrome. This condition is actually a range of developmental irregularities in the eye due to unusual separation of the anterior segment tissues. It happens in the embryonic growth of the eye. These include posterior embryotoxon, Axenfeld syndrome, Rieger's anomaly, Reiger syndrome and Peters syndrome.

Corneal opacities, present at birth – Injury, present at birth glaucoma, infection, Peters syndrome, present at birth inherited abnormal development in the endothelium (both recessive and dominant types), present at birth inherited abnormal development of the stroma and mucopolysaccharidosis.

Glaucoma

Glaucoma in a child, is frequently present at birth and marked with irregular growth of the trabecular meshwork elements that go on to be swelling and fluid in the cornea and large eyeballs in the infant. The patient may experience watery eyes, light sensitivity, blepharospasm, swelling and fluid in the cornea, a cornea that is bigger than normal and unusually large eyeballs. The inheritance is autosomal recessive (particularly for Middle Eastern areas). The majority of cases are influenced by more than one gene and more than one factor. Identify the condition early. Assess the person with anesthesia and give particular care to check the IOP, measurements of the cornea, gonioscopy, optic nerve assessment and A-scan biometry. Try to clean up the cornea by getting the IOP down with beta-blockers, carbonic anhydrase inhibitors in the body and on the skin and prostaglandin inhibitors. The ultimate medical attention is an operation.

The person will need habitual check-ups (with anesthesia). Aid lazy eye, nearsightedness and eye misalignment. Similar symptoms may indicate nasolacrimal duct block, present at birth megalocornea or present at birth inherited abnormal development in the endothelium.

Conditions linked to glaucoma - Anterior segment faulty development, posterior embryotoxon, Axenfeld's anomaly, Rieger's anomaly, Reiger syndrome, Peter's anomaly. It is linked to any syndrome linked to present at birth glaucoma, including Sturge-Weber syndrome, Lowe syndrome, Rubinstein-Taybi syndrome, neurofibromatosis trisomy 13, abnormally small eyeballs, coloboma, and cataract and growth abnormality in the retina. Glaucoma is linked secondary glaucoma, including aphakic glaucoma, German measles, bleeding inside the eye, juvenile rheumatoid arthritis, juvenile xanthogranuloma, retinoblastoma, retinopathy of prematurity and displacement of the lens of the eye.

Lens Disorders

Coloboma - Focal notch or abnormality on the lens. It is caused by the lack of or interruption of zonules at the time the lens is forming. You may see focal flattening or notch, elongated or lack of zonules next to the problem and another form of coloboma in the iris, ciliary body or elsewhere.

Cataracts in one eye, present at birth - Sometimes is has no known cause, other times it is due to persistent hyperplastic primary vitreous, injury or faulty development of the anterior segment.

Microspherophakia - Lens which is irregularly sphere-shaped. It is more likely to become misplaced to the anterior. You may see a lens that is little and curved, misplaced towards the anterior, obstruction in the pupillary area and a resulting problem with glaucoma. This condition is linked to Weill-Marchesani syndrome, a problem that includes an undersized physique and squat fingers.

Congenital subluxation or dislocation of the lens - Generally arises due to feeble zonules. You may see partial dislocation of the lens, partial dislocation in the inferonasal area, partial dislocation of the superotemporal area and elongated or busted zonular fibers. In the body, you may find Marfan syndrome or homocystinuria.

Cataracts in both eyes, present at birth - No known cause, inherited, or disease in the body which may include Lowe syndrome, galactosemia, Alport syndrome, Down syndrome, myotonic muscle disorder, Fabry's disease or Wilson's disease. The problem may also be due to toxoplasmosis, German measles present at birth, cytomegalovirus, HSV, varicella-zoster virus, syphilis, malformation of the anterior segment or lack of an iris.

Congenital cataracts - May arise due to problems during fetal growth of the lens. In both eyes, many times it is due to an irregularity of the body. This is a sign that a body workup is needed to identify the reason. To assess, check titers for toxoplasmosis, rubella, cytomegalovisur, HSV or another form of present at birth syphilis or virus. Check for syphilis. Do urine analysis. When the opacity is insignificant and does not alter the person's sight, it is okay to postpone the cataract operation pending the person getting older. Medical attention may include taking out the cataract and not putting in a lens into the eye, then using aphakic contact lenses. Putting an intraocular lens into a baby or child is debatable and still being researched. Similar symptoms may indicate leukoma in the cornea, coloboma, retinoblastoma, another form of tumor in the eye, infection, endophthalmitis, separation of the retina or PHVP.

Uveitis

Pediatric uveitis - May be caused by an autoimmune problem such as juvenile rheumatoid arthritis, sarcoid, HLA-B27 or no known cause. It may be due to an infection such as toxocariasis, aftermath of viral inflammation of the retina and optic nerve, Lyme disease, HSV, HZV, TB, Syphilis or cytomegalovirus. It may be due to a masquerade syndrome such as retinoblastoma, lymphoma, foreign body inside the eye, juvenile xanthogranuloma or injury.

Juvenile rheumatoid arthritis-linked uveitis – Ongoing inflammation in the anterior that is frequently seen in females who are not yet 16 years old. It includes oligoarticular or pauciarticular arthritis, negative rheumatoid factor and positive antinuclear antibody. Many times it is made more complex because of cystoid swelling and fluid in the macula and band corneal dystrophy. The problem has no known cause. The patient may experience fuzzy sight, moving dark spots in vision, or some people do not experience any indications in the eyes and may only find the problem following an unsuccessful sight test or leukocoria due to fully developed cataract. Similar symptoms may indicate sarcoid eye inflammation, psoriatic arthritis, Lyme disease, flare-up of bowel disease, HSV, HZV or injury. 113.4 instances of JRA for every 100,000 kids. Half are pauciarticular or oligoarticular, and of these 20% get eye inflammation. Girls get JRA more, 5:1. When JRA sets in prior to the time the child is 6 years old there is more of a danger of eye inflammation arising. You may see nongranulomatous eye inflammation in the anterior of one eye in the beginning, and 75% of people will have the other eye affected. Usually the conjunctiva is fine. You may find band corneal dystrophy, cataract, adhesion of the pupil to the lens, glaucoma, cystoid swelling and fluid in the macula and shrinking of the eyeball. Medical attention includes steroids on the skin or eyelid unless there is ongoing flare. Continue watching and managing any eye difficulties that arise. Check for lazy eye. Do cataract operation to keep lazy eye from occurring. Do not put lens into the eye. Refractory flare-up could necessitate steroids taken by mouth or immunosuppressive agents. Drugs used include mydriatics and steroids.

Intermediate uveitis – Fibroglial cells and strocytes show up on top of the periphery of the retina. Lymphocytes can be on the peripheral retina and going into the walls of the blood vessels in the retina. There is eventual arising of flare-up of the anterior vitreous, linked to slight nongranulomatous anterior chamber flare-up, peripheral inflamed blood vessels in the retina, vitreous opacities, snow banks and CME. It has no known cause. The patient may experience moving gaps in vision and lessened sight. It accounts for ¼ of every instance of pediatric uveitis. ¾ of people have it in both eyes. You may find anterior chamber cells and flare, adhesion of the pupil to the lens, band corneal dystrophy, peripheral inflamed blood vessels, snow balls/snow banks, too many vessels in the retina, separation of the retina, glaucoma and CME. To assess, use fluorescein x-ray of blood vessels, chest x-ray, MRI when there could be multiple sclerosis and an assessment for Lyme disease.

Steroids on the skin or lids along with mydriatics in the beginning. Immunosuppression in the body could become needed if the condition is refractive. People need to have habitual assessments for lazy eye, glaucoma and CME. Pars plana cold therapy and surgical removal of the vitreous are needed in some cases when the person's case is significant. Drugs include steroids (skin, lid and by mouth), mydriatic agents, and immunosuppressents in the body. Similar symptoms may indicate sarcoid, toxocariasis, peripheral toxoplasmosis, foreign body in the eye, lyme disease or TB.

Toxocariasis

Toxocariasis is in one eye, posterior pole or peripheral nodules of inflammatory cells and inflammation of the vitreous body. It is seen in children, with the average age seven-and-a-half when the problem shows up. It is caused by *T. canis* larvae when a child eats the eggs. The patient may experience lessened sight in one eye, moving gaps in sight, light sensitivity, a case that is between acute and chronic and a case that looks a lot like retinoblastoma. You may also find optic nerve disorder in some cases, tractional separation of the retina, glaucoma and cataract. Other symptoms in the body include high body temperature, difficulty breathing, enlarged liver, neurological problems and finding that the larvae in the eye are not alive anymore. Assessments include enzyme-associated immunosorbent assay for the organism. Check for a raised peripheral blood eosinophil amount.

Make sure it is not another infection in the body. Larvae that is not alive is believed as more immunogenic than larvae that is alive. Eye flare-up can become greater once anihelmintic therapy has been done. In the beginning, use steroids in the body or lids. Surgical removal of the vitreous may be needed in some cases. Drugs include thiabendazole and prednisone. Similar symptoms may indicate retinoblastoma, toxoplasmosis, primary hyperplastic vitreous, Coats' disease, sarcoid or ROP.

PHPV

Persistent hyperplastic primary vitreous (PHPV) ranges widely in how bad the condition gets and may include front or back and have a range of vascularization. Generally there is fibrous plaque at the posterior lens capsule and unrelenting hyaloid elements that go back in the direction of the optic nerve. It is present at birth as an irregularity in the eye due to the main vitreous not reverting. The patient may experience a little eye, white pupil, eye misalignment, quick and involuntary movements of the eye and lessened sight. You will see it in one eye. There is an anterior chamber that is not as deep as normal, ciliary procedures are moved towards the middle into blood vessel filled fibrovascular membrane, raised IOP, fibrovascular stalk that begins at the back of the lens and goes to the optic nerve and cataract. Use ultrasound to assess. When there is no medical attention, the problem may worsen to become cataract, pupil obstruction, cyclitic membrane, glaucoma, separation of the retina, and slow wasting away. Medical attention includes surgical removal of the lens, membrane or anterior vitreous, help for the absence of the natural lens and treatment for lazy eye.

ROP

Retinopathy of prematurity (ROP), also called retrolental fibrosis happens in babies born prematurely; irregular neovascularization in the retina arises at the meeting point of developed and underdeveloped retina. This creates cicatrix alterations such as traction in the macula, separation in the retina or wasting away. There are many elements that create the problem. Mainly it is thought that for the underdeveloped retina, too much oxygen causes vasoconstriction and the inferior problem of a lack of oxygen in the retina, freedom of blood vessel development elements and development of new blood vessels. This condition is also linked to how much the baby weighs at birth, gestational age, oxygen, infection in the blood, replacing the baby's blood, bleeding in ventricles, necrotizing enterocolitis and abnormal development of bronchopulmonary area.

ROP worsens from stage 1 to stage 5, but it can heal on its own during any one of the stages. Ongoing cicatrix alterations with this condition may be no vascularization in the periphery, folding in the retina, macula that has moved towards the temporal area, alteration in the pigment of the epithelium, traction or rhegmatogenous separation of the retina.

Any baby lighter than 1500g or who is 34 weeks in gestational age needs to be checked for this condition. The baby needs to be checked when he reaches 32 weeks' gestational age, then checked again every two weeks pending the development of the retina. When the condition is in zone 1 or 2, check the area every week. A baby with small weight at birth has a higher chance of getting this condition. Similar symptoms may indicate familial exudative vitreoretinopathy, Coats' disease, posterior persistent hyperplastic primary vitreous or toxocariasis.

Medical attention for ROP includes cold therapy or circuitous ophthalmoscopically given laser treatments to the retina with no blood vessels if the patient has threshold disease (according to Cryo-ROP study). This can stop it from worsening. It might make the condition go away and can stop it causing lessened sight in the future. Someone who has had it has more chance of eye misalignment or needing lenses for nearsightedness or astigmatism. The child needs habitual checkups until the 5th birthday.

ROP is classified in terms of the zones of location, including zones 1,2 and 3, the amount of disease that there is which is depicted by hours on the "clock" of the retina, and stages of the disease, including:

- Stage 1 – demarcation line
- Stage 2 – ridge
- Stage 3 – ridge and fibrovascular spreading in the extraretinal area
- Stage 4 – subtotal separation of the retina, including 4A (extrafoveal) and 4B (separation of the retina and the fovea)
- Stage 5 – complete separation of the retina
- Plus disease – vascular enlargement and twisting

Threshold disease – 5 or more adjacent clock hours or 8 total clock hours with stage 3 of this condition and located in zone 1 or 2 along with Plus disease.

Coats' Disease and Wagner Syndrome

Coats' disease – Present at birth telangectasia in the retina that causes exudative separation in the retina. It is generally in one eye in a male child (age 8). The patient may experience eye misalignment, lessened sight and white pupil. You may see aneurismal enlargement and telangiectasia in the blood vessels of the retina, exudation in the subretina, exudative separation of the retina and cholesterol crystals in the subretina. Left with no medical attention, the separation in the retina could cause the neovascular goaucoma and shrunken eye. Medical attention includes cold therapy or laser treatment on the irregular vessels. This might stop exudation and worsening for the condition. Similar symptoms indicate retinoblastoma, toxocariasis, retinopathy of prematurity and familial exudative vitreoretinopathy.

Wagner syndrome – Inherited autosomal dominant; abnormal development of vitreoretinal area that causes medium amount nearsightedness (-3 to -4D) and irregularities in the vitreoretinal area. There is unusual collagen production.

Vitreous is not full, degeneration in the vitreous, separation of the vitreous in the back, peripheral blood vessel sheathing, and early creation of cataract. The condition is much like Stickler syndrome, but it has less of a chance of separation of the retina and preventative laser treatment is not encouraged. Take out cataract if it is affecting sight. Use the correct refraction and check for any fractures or rips in the retina.

Vitreoretinal Dysplasia

Vitreoretinal dysplasia is acollection of conditions having to do with poor growth in the retina and vitreous, including vitreoretinal abnormal development, incontinentia pigmenti, Warburg syndrome and trisomy 13. They can happen by themselves or together with other bodily problems. Do hereditary analysis abnormal development in the retina and linked bodily problems. A number of hereditary investigations have been recognized for some types of abnormal development of the retina. The problem worsens to significant lessening of sight. Medical attention includes managing poor sight. Similar symptoms indicate ROP, retinoblastoma, astrocytic hamartoma, retinal separation and familial exudative vitreoretinopathy.

Stickler Syndrome

Stickler syndrome is inherited autosomal dominant with the fault in procollagen II gene; marked with a lot of nearsightedness, separation of the retina, marked features on the face and joint disease that worsens with time. You may see nearsightedness that is more than -8D, transparent vitreous including strands and veils, separation of the retina, glaucoma, nuclear cataracts in the sclera, opaque places in the cortex, and perivscular pigmentation. The problem is a fault in collagen cell growth that creates irregularities in the bone, vitreous and retina. The myopia can commonly create giant rips in the retina and a number of fractures in the retina. The patient will also have cataracts develop which worsen with time. Medical attention includes vitreoretinal operation to manage fractures in the retina and preventative laser treatment on the places where the retina is becoming thin. Continue watchful check-ups to look for disease in the retina arising. Similar symptoms may indicate Wagner syndrome.

Goldmann-Favre Disease

Goldmann-Favre disease is an autosomal recessive; retinoschisis in the retina and fovea including syneresis of the vitreous. The patient will experience progressive lessening of sight and eventual inability to see at night. You may see syneresis in the vitreous including strands and veils, degeneration in the vitreous and fovea, wasting away of the pigment in the peripheral retina, darkening of the peripheral retina with an inflammation of the retina pigmentosa type design, , blood vessel sheathing in the periphery and less than normal ERG. Check ERG and EOG for irregularities. Check sight. In the early years, cataracts may form. With time, the retina's function gets worse and ERG readings are lessened. Retinoschisis needs to be carefully observed since the retina can fracture as an added problem. Similar symptoms may indicate abnormal development of the cone or RP.

Familial Exudative Vitreoretinopathy

Familial exudative vitreoretinopathy (FEVR) is an autosomal dominant; gradual worsening of vitroretinopathy which causes traction in the retina and in the back of the vitreous. When the vessels have traction there may be escape of liquids and alteration in the color of the epithelium as an added issue. It is linked to irregularities Norrie's disease. Hereditary assessments show a shared trail for Norrie's and FEVR. You may see fibrovascular spreading in the periphery of the retina including traction, traction that is linked to enlarged tortuous blood vessels and fluid coming out all around, traction that worsens with time to become complete separation of the retina, and cataract and neovascular glaucoma as additional problems. Under a microscope, the alterations are much like the ones demonstrated with cicatricial ROP. Medical attention includes cold therapy or circuitous laser treatment on the area that is not getting enough blood flow in the periphery of the retina to stop the ongoing traction. Check kids who have problems in the macula or fovea for poor sight.

Retinoschisis and Retinitis

Juvenile X-linked retinoschisis - Occurs in male children (ages 5 to 10); marked with retinoschisis in the fovea. The patient may experience lessened sight, half have retinoschisis in the periphery, half have vitreous veils, bleeding and degeneration, and alterations in the periphery of the retina such as sheathing around the blood vessels. Do ERG and EOG to assess. Under a miscroscope, samples show cuts in the nerve fiber layer. With time, the problem will have very gradual lessening in the middle of sight (but may be finger counting for some people), progression to total-thickness punctures in the retina and bleeding vitreous. Medical attention for the punctures will be necessary. Similar symptoms may indicate Goldmann-Favre disease, Stickler syndrome or Wagner syndrome.

Retinitis punctate albescens – Type of retinitis pigmentosa; marked with many white spots all through the retina. It is autosomal recessive. Patient indications and medical attention compares to RP. You may see weakened vessels, pale disc and white spots. This is a gradually worsening condition but the central sight is saved into the 50's.

Retinitis pigmentosa – Collection of conditions marked with ongoing worsening of abnormal rod development and cones that are not as badly influenced. Usually there is worsening ability to see at night, lessened field of vision and irregular ERG records. It can be autosomal dominant, autosomal recessive or X-associated recessive. When it is recessive or X-associated, it generally starts earlier and gets worse faster than the autosomal dominant type. The patient may also gave alterations in the field of vision that start as gaps in sight and worsen to become just a little middle spot of sight. You may see weak blood vessels in the retina, wasting away in the epithelium in the beginning that moves on to be traditional pigment sediment and creation of bone spicule as time goes by, waxy paleness in the optic disc, cloudy places in the vitreous, cataracts, fluid and swelling in the macula and wasting away in the macula as the later phases occur.

Medical attention includes doing an ERG, find out inheritance, check dark adjustment curves and field of vision. Progressed instances have a great deal of lessening of rods and cones. Medical attention includes management with diet to stop worsening with Refsum's disease and abetalipoproteinemia. Adding vitamin A to the diet can stop worsening of retrophysiologic alterations. Identifying the problem early and getting proper advice is vital for finding out if particular instructional requirements will be needed in a child with this condition. Use tinted lenses to aid problems with adjusting to the dark. Swelling and fluid in the macula can be handled with steroids on the lid or acetazolamide taken by mouth. Similar symptoms of inability to see at night may indicate present at birth stationary inability to see at night, fundus albipunctatus, choideremia or lack of vitamin A. Similar symptoms of pigmentary disease in the retina may indicate injury, present at birth infection, toxicity due to drug, serous separation of the retina that has been treated.

Fundus Albipunctatus

Fundus albipunctatus is an autosomal recessive type of stable inability to see at night marked with white spots all through the retina. You may see scattered white spots on the same plane as the pigment epithelium. The macula is not generally affected. There is no paleness in the optic nerve and the vessels are not weakened. Do ERG to find lessened scotopic B wave and significantly postponed dark adjustment. Sight stays fine. Similar symptoms may indicate fleck abnormal development of the retina.

Night Blindness and Achromkatopsia

Congenital stationary night blindness – Present at birth, lessened sight, nearsightedness and no problem in the fundus. It is autosomal dominant, autosomal recessive or X-associated. If dominant, the sight is usually fine. Otherwise the sight in the central area is lessened. Recessive or X-associated types are linked to nearsightedness, quick and involuntary movement in the eyes, eye misalignment and contradictory pupil reactions. Do ERG. The inability to see at night will be static, but the nearsightedness might worsen with time. There is no medical attention. Similar symptoms may indicate Oguchi's disease.

Congenital achromatopsia – (rod monochromatism) – Present at birth and does not worsen with time. It is marked with a lack of useful cones and indications of lessened sight in the center, total inability to differentiate colors, quick and involuntary movements in the eyes and light sensitivity. It is autosomal recessive. With low light, the ability to see gets a lot better. High refractive errors are commonly seen, but the fundus is fine. Sight may be lessened to 20/200. Do ERG, dark adjustment curve, check color sight and pupil responses. As time goes by, nystagmus has a propensity for diminishing amplitude and frequency. Sight is lessened from the time of birth but does not worsen with time. Medical attention includes utilizing dark lenses. Similar symptoms may indicate some achromatopsia, partial rod monochromatism or blue cone monochromatism.

Dystrophies and Flavimaculatus

Fleck dystrophies – Collection of hereditary conditions which have yellow or white accumulations all through the retina.

Fundus flavimaculatus, or Stargardt's disease – Autosomal recessive; fish-shaped or fishtail-shaped flecks all through the retina. The patient have lessened sight in the middle. The condition might be hard to identify in the beginning since flecks can be hard to see. You may see the flecks through the posterior pole, lessened middle foveal reflex, bull's-eye maculopathy, hammered-metal look in the macula and lessened ability to see (20/200). Use fluorescein x-ray. ERG/EOG will be standard.

Best's vitelliform dystrophy – Ages 4 to 10, autosomal dominant, large range of measurable characteristics. This condition does include a cyst-like element that is a shade of yellow/orange in the macula. It has stages from 0 to 4. A fundus that is fine is stage 0. Stage 2 is standard vitelliform lesion. Stage 3 looks like pseudohypopyon. Stage 4 has wasting away in the macula or fibrotic scar. Do EOP. Worsening is different for each person. Sometimes it goes to stage 4, sometimes it has lessened sight and the majority still have useful sight during the lifespan.

Nerve Disorders

Optic disc coloboma – Present at birth pit in the optic disc due to unfinished shutting of embryonic fissure. There are no tendencies for certain ethnicities or male/female, but there have been instances of more than one case in a family. The patient may experience eye misalignment and lessened sight from slight to significant (contingent upon the papillomacular bundle being affected or not). The pit is shaped like a bowl and generally in the inferior. The choroid next to it can become affected. When it goes further than the optic nerve, the eye will commonly be microphthalmic. When it is in the optic disc, it is commonly in both eyes. The problem may worsen to become retinal separation. Handle that with photocoagulation or surgical removal of the vitreous. It could heal on its own in some cases. Optic nerve coloboma is treated with patches to aid lazy eye. Similar symptoms may indicate morning glory disc irregularity.

This condition might be linked to another coloboma in the iris, ciliary body or retina. This condition is seen with a number of other syndromes, including coloboma, heart disease, choanal atresia, slow growth, genital irregularity, ear irregularity or hard of hearing, Walker-Warburg syndrome, Acardia syndrome, Goldenhar's sequence, linear sebaceous nevus syndrome and Goltz focal dermal hypoplasia.

Optic nerve hypoplasia – Present at birth, little and underdeveloped optic nerve head; linked to irregular peripapillary pigmentation and irregular blood vessel design. Commonly linked to endocrinologic irregularities. It has no known cause, but may be due to main failure to axons to grow or excessive programmed cell death. It is linked to the mom using teratogenic agents or to maternal diabetes. The patient may experience noteworthy optic nerve underdevelopment in both eyes, quick and involuntary eye movements, lessened sight and eye misalignment. A meek case could just have a bit of lessened sight and irregular field of vision. Most instances are random, but it has been seen in families.

Optic pits – Scattered, circular, pit in the optic disc that is a shade of gray/white and generally in the temporal region. It could be a slight case of optic nerve coloboma or it may be a regional fault in how the nerve and retinal pigment epithelium grew. It is not linked to serous macular separation. The sight should be fine and have no indications. It is generally in one eye, although it does happen in both eyes for 15% of people. The pit ranges in measurements. 25%-75% of eyes also get serous macular separation that lessens the ability to see. The pits have protrusions of abnormally developed retina including faults in the lamina cribrosa. Sometimes there is contact from the vitreous cavity and the subretinal or subarachnoid area. Tend to serous separation with surgical removal of the vitreous or photocoagulation. Similar symptoms may indicate optic nerve coloboma or morning glory disc irregularity.

Morning glory optic nerve anomaly – Present at birth, formed like a funnel, pit in the optic disc and posterior fundus. It is a fault from the embryo development. Patient may experience lessened ability to see from 20/200 to hand movements and eye misalignment. It is seen in girls more than boys (very unusual in African American children). The cases are generally random. You may see it in one eye with a bigger than normal disc, funnel-like pit, white clump of glial tissue in the middle of the disc, vascularity from the borders of the disc instead of from the middle and a balanced pit all the way in a circle. It is frequently linked to transphenoidal type of basal encephalocele. Use MRI to make sure it is not encephalocele. Some people get serous retinal separation (40%) in addition. Medical attention includes patching to handle lazy eye and aid sight. Similar symptoms may indicate optic nerve coloboma or optic nerve pit.

Myelinated nerve fibers – White patchy lines on the retina of oligodendrocytes and myelin inside the retina. It is believed to be a fault in lamina cribrosa letting the oligodendrocytes move within the eye and by the nerve fiber layer so that myelinization can occur. Unless it is in one eye, it is linked to nearsightedness. The majority retain good sight and do not have indications. It happens for up to 1% of all people, and 20% have it in both eyes. Up to 20% look intermittent from the optic nerve head. You may see the far end shaped like a fan and going along the nerve fiber layer. The blood vessels in the retina are blocked by myelination. It is found with Gorlin-Goltz syndrome, may be autosomal dominant, or when it is in one eye it is linked to a lot of nearsightedness and lazy eye. This last category generally does not respond to occlusion treatment and cannot get good sight. Similar symptoms may indicate papilledema or retina inflammation.

Optic nerve hypoplasia – Present at birth, little and underdeveloped optic nerve head; linked to irregular peripapillary pigmentation and irregular blood vessel design. Commonly linked to endocrinologic irregularities. It has no known cause, but may be due to main failure to axons to grow or excessive programmed cell death. It is linked to the mom using teratogenic agents or to maternal diabetes. The patient may experience noteworthy optic nerve underdevelopment in both eyes, quick and involuntary eye movements, lessened sight and eye misalignment. A meek case could just have a bit of lessened sight and irregular field of vision. Most instances are random, but it has been seen in families.

You may see unusually little optic nerve and just a slight bit of yellow/pink tissue from the optic nerve. The region around has exposed sclera and a band of retinal pigment epithelium on the border of it. This white sclera may be mistaken for regular tissue from the retina. You will see tortuous blood vessels in the retina. Sight can be 20/20 to no ability to see light. Sight is not related to measurement of optic nerve. People frequently have astigmatism. The condition is linked to CNS irregularities and septooptic dysplasia. Do MRI to make sure there is not an irregularity in the hypothalamic pituitary axis. The condition of the optic nerve is stable in the lifespan, but neuroendocrine irregularities can arise as time goes by. Try occlusion treatment to handle lazy eye.

Treat problems of astigmatism. Recommend a low-vision specialist as soon as possible. Similar symptoms may indicate optic nerve coloboma, optic nerve pit or wasting away in the optic nerve.

Optic nerve atrophy – Marked by paleness in optic disc due to disease that results in the ganglion cell axons dying in the retina including compressive abnormal optic nerve functioning, compressive lesion affecting bone, toxic optic wasting away, injury related abnormal optic nerve functioning, neurodegenerative irregularities, extensive harm to the retina, or no known cause. The patient may experience lessened sight, harm to optic nerve beginning in babyhood can cause quick and involuntary eye movements, see-saw quick and involuntary eye movements, pulled back eyelid and setting-sun indication, nystagmus along with nodding head, feebleness, loss of coordination or focal neurologic problems. Another form of neurologic indication can aid in finding the pressing lesion. Take a thorough account of family medical records because it may be inherited. You may see that the sight goes along with the amount of wasting away, broad paleness in the optic disc, afferent pupillary fault, lessened ability to see contrasts, and present at birth lesions can create transsynaptic deterioration and more wasting away in the optic nerve heads.

Get a neurologist, do MRI and assess color sight. The progression is contingent upon the reason for the optic atrophy. This condition could show up as long as 6 weeks following harm, so sequential check-ups are needed to see if the problem is stable or worsening. Similar symptoms may indicate optic nerve hypoplasia or present at birth optic nerve irregularity.

Leber's hereditary optic atrophy – Medical attention includes instructing the patient to stop using alcohol and to stop smoking since these may worsen the problem Similar symptoms may indicate ischemic optic neuropathy, tobacco/alcohol lazy eye, MS or dominant optic atrophy.

Periocular swelling and proptosis – Similar symptoms may indicate preseptal or orbital cellulitis, orbital pseudotumor, leukemia, optic nerve glioma, neurofibroma, rhabdomyosarcoma or neuroblastoma.

Leber's hereditary optic atrophy – Hard to identify until the condition is established, both eyes have optic neuropathy due to a problem in mitochondrial DNA. It is hereditary from the mother and linked to a number of mitochondrial DNA irregularities. It is frequently a problem with nucleotide alterations on location 11778 and other mutations affecting locations 3460, 14482, 15257 and 4160. It shows up from 15 to 30 years old in one eye. The patient may experience fuzzy sight which may lessen to 20/200. The other eye may be affected after days or months. It is more frequently found in males (9:1) in the United States. Outside of the U.S. there is a 50%-80% tendency for it to be in men. You may see circumpapillary telangiectatic microangiopathy, pseudopapilledema in the disc and no seeping from the fluorescein x-ray. A number of people could also have heart irregularities, so EKG and Holter assessment may be done. Do hereditary analysis to see if the genes are altered.

Dominant optic atrophy (Kjer type) – majority of inherited wasting away of the optic nerve problems fall into this category. It is hard to identify until the condition has become well established. There is lessened sight in initial 10 years (20/70 to 20/100 as a final result). This condition is matched to chromosome 3 (3q28-qter). The patient experiences lessened sight as seen during a regular check-up, and frequently there is also slight light sensitivity. You may see paleness in the temporal part of the optic nerve. Lessened nerve fiber layer may be demonstrated with red-free filtering when you look at the papillomacular bundle. Check color sight to find a problem with blue/yellow recognition. Field of vision should be regular. Research shows that the problem is main deterioration in the ganglion cells of the retina. Sight begins to lessen at age 4 to 6, then it worsens gradually during the next twenty years. Hereditary analysis is needed. Similar symptoms may indicate Leber's optic neuropathy or optic neuropathy with no known cause.

Behr's optic atrophy – Autosomal recessive wasting away linked to another neurological irregularity such as loss of coordination, lessened muscle tone or lessened mental ability. It arises from age 1 to 9 and the neurological indications worsen with time along with significant wasting away in the optic area. It is equally found in males and females. It is in both eyes, and half also get quick and involuntary eye movements. Check MRI for white matter irregularities. The patient may also have irregular metabolic functions. There is no medical attention. Similar symptoms may indicate Leber's optic neuropathy or dominant optic atrophy.

Capillary hemangioma – Benign growth in periocular tissue that is there at birth and quickly get bigger in the initial 6 months of the lifespan. There are two ways that they show up.

1. It may grow outward as a strawberry lesion including elevated, asymmetrical growths on the skin.
2. It may be a deep growth so that the conjunctiva and periocular tissue are a shade of blue.

Periorbital Infections

Preseptal cellulitis – Eyelid infection and infection around the eyes in front of orbital septum. It can be transferred from regional hordeola, adjacent to infection in the sinus and linked to upper respiratory tract infection, or due to injury. The eyelids will be puffy and red. The patient may have prior skin injury or sinus infection. You may see swelling and fluid and redness in the lids, total movement around the eye, no hurting during eye activity and swelling and fluid around the eye. The eye does not bulge out of the socket. Medical attention includes antibiotics in the body, watching the case to make sure it is getting better in a day or two, and CT or MRI if the puffiness is not getting better quickly.

Do study of tissue sample to see chubby endothelial cells. After the initial 6 to 8 months, it stops growing. Subsequently, the problem eventually mends during the next 4-5 years. Similar symptoms may indicate rhabdomyosarcoma, orbital cellulitis, pyogenic granuloma, chalazion or hordeola.

Orbital cellulitis – Soft tissue infection in back of the septum of the orbit. It may be due to infection that has spread (sinus, dental, lacrimal sac), injury, or it may be produced by the body as bacteria in the bloodstream. You may see lessened action around the eye, lessened sight, significant and irregular pupillary reactions, bulging eye, inflamed conjunctiva and inflamed and red eyelid. The person may be septic with bacteria in the bloodstream. Use CT to make sure it is not abscesses. Do cultures on fluid to look at bacteria and fungi. Medical attention includes going to the hospital for antibiotics into the veins and getting the fluid out of infected sinus or abscess areas.

Inflammatory orbital pseudotumor – Bulging eyeball out of the socket and flare-up in periocular area; lack of septis; lack of infection. There may also be inflammation of pappila and iris. papillitis and iris. Use CT or MRI. Medical attention includes large dosage of corticosteroids. Biopsy may be needed when it is not getting better quickly.

Capillary Hemangioma

Capillary hemangioma are growths on the eyelid and periocular area. Sight might be affected with lazy eye because of block or provoked astigmatism. There is a tendency for periocular area, head and neck. Big tumors could create low platelet count by isolation of the platelets. A hemangioma on the periocular tissue necessitates quick assessment of the whole body to see what other areas are affected (some of which may result in heart problems). Scattered capillary hemangiomatosis may be linked to heart issues and could create blocked airways. Medical attention includes observation to see if lazy eye arises, occlusion treatment to correct lazy eye, and corticosteroids for blocking amblyopia or noteworthy astigmatism. Intralesional injections are shown to be linked to regional complications such as focal necrosis and skin discoloration. Corticosteroids given into the vein may cause secondary clotting in ophthalmic artery and cause a block in the artery of the middle retina. Carefully watch lazy eye. Steroids can give a quick ricochet experience and lesion may get bigger when decreasing the steroids.

Lymphangioma

Lymphangioma is a benign orbital tumor in conjunctiva, lid or orbit; contains fluid and causes abrupt bulging eyeball (by age 6). The patient may have eye misalignment when the mass moves in on the muscles outside the eye. It is present at birth and gradually gets bigger. There may be unprompted bleeding (chocolate cyst) which causes abrupt eye bulging, heightened IOP, hurting and subconjunctiva bleeding. When bleeding goes away, the bulging may go away on its own. A respiratory tract infection may cause more indications. Do MRI or CT. These tumors are big, full of serum cysts that are lined with flat endothelial cells. Lymphoid tissue could be all through the interstitium. Use glaucoma drugs and decompression for the cyst (by draining the blood out) for bulging and raised IOP. Open biopsy may be done. The use of debulking is restricted to instances of bleeding which does not get better on its own or to cases of noteworthy bulging and eye misalignment. Similar symptoms may indicate orbital hemangioma, rhabdomyosarcoma or orbital pseudotumor.

Rhabdomyosarcoma

Rhabdomyosarcoma is a malignant orbital tumor most frequently seen orbit malignancy during childhood; frequently seen as quickly worsening eye bulging out of the socket. Patient may experience inflammation in the eyelids and a mass that can be felt by touch. The eye may have redness which does not go away with antibiotics. Frequently there has been preceding injury. Do CT or MRI, biopsy as soon as possible and give sample for electron miscroscopy and immunohistochemical stains. The prediction for the future used to be bad, but now chemotherapy and radiation are used. People who have radiation have more of a chance of keratoconjunctivitis, provoked cataract, radiation abnormal optic nerve function and radiation disease of the retina. Similar symptoms may indicate orbital cellulitis, hemangioma, lymphangioma, neuroblastoma or metastatic retinoblastoma.

Retinoblastoma - habitual check-ups are needed with anesthesia. Habitual check-ups from a pediatric oncologist and neurologist need to be done as well. Similar symptoms may indicate inflammation, another type of tumor, irregular growth, inherited disease or more.

Forms of Rhabdomyosarcoma:

- Embryonal – Most frequently seen, coming from mesenchymal tissue with no specialized function located in the orbit. The majority of cases are in the superonasal quadrant.
- Alveolar – Worst in terms of prediction for the future of these four forms; frequently affects inferior orbit.
- Pleomorphic – Least often seen; best prediction for the future; most specialized
- Botryoid – Is only seen as a secondary expansion from paranasal sinus area

Orbital Tumors

Neuroblastoma -- Metastatic orbital tumor most frequently seen metastatic tumor of the orbit for children; does not hurt, worsening with time bulging of the eyeball out of the socket and commonly found with bruised eyelid. It spreads from the abdomen with sympathetic or parasympathetic chains. It generally begins at approximately age 2. Eye bulging occurs quickly, there are lytic bone lesions, and 40% have it in both eyes. Use urine vanillylmandelic acid assessment (which will be raised). Medical attention includes chemotherapy and radiation. Prediction for the future is bad.

Optic nerve glioma – Most frequently seen inferior quality pilocytic nervous system tumor that grows from astrocytes; most frequently seen optic nerve tumor for kids. It does not hurt, has bulging of the eye from the socket, lessened central vision, lessened ability to see color, and chiasmal glioma will also have lessened sight in both eyes. It generally begins before age 10, and girls get it more often than boys. It is linked to optic nerve glioma and neurofibromatosis. Around 15% of kids who have neurofibromatosis also get this condition. 1/3 of kids who have this condition also have neurofibrosis. The patient experiences a gap in the middle of the sight field, wasting away in the optic area, optociliary shunt vessels, wasting away in the band may be found in chiasmal glioma, and quick beginning of glioma could occur along with puffy and fluid-filled optic nerve. Similar symptoms may indicate nerve sheath hemangioma, schwannoma, craniopharyngioma or eosinophilic granuloma.

Do CT or MRI. Someone who has neurofibromatosis type I could also get another eye indication such as plexiform neuroma in the lid, lack of sphenoid wing, Lisch nodes or café-au-lait areas. It may affect in the pituitary and create endocrine irregularities. Use endocrinologic assessment when the person has chiasmal or suprasellar issues. The medical attention for this condition is debatable. A number of people believe they are benign hamartomatous lesions including noteworthy cases with extended lack of visible activity or getting better on its own. These people encourage conservative treatment. Chiasmal problems usually get worse quicker and move to hypothalamus or third ventricle. This can create blocked hydrocephalus. When the patient has slight lessened sight, watch the case. Worsening sight might necessitate radiation. Big tumors that develop fast may necessitate an incision into the orbit and cutting it out. Chiasmal glioma needs radiation treatment. Watch the patient after treatment and check sight, field of vision and sequential imaging to watch how the tumor develops.

Meningioma – For a kid, it can affect the orbit coming in from meninges in the optic nerve sheath or coming in from sphenoid wing. This condition is spreading meningothelial cells that generally begin in the optic nerve sheath. The patient may experience bulging eyeball, lessened sight and eye misalignment. You may also find wasting away in the optic nerve and optociliary shunt vessels located in the optic disc. Do MRI or CT. The problem is gradually worsening but does not spread. Watch the case closely. Cutting it out does not usually mend the problem and could actually make sight worse. Cutting it out and radiation treatment could be used when the problem continues to worsen. Similar symptoms may indicate optic nerve glioma.

Retinoblastoma – Most frequently seen malignant tumor in the eye for kids; seen in 1/20,000 babies born alive. Two types include inherited and not inherited. The inherited form is caused by genetic lack in chromosome 13q14. The not hereditary type happens when two mutational events happen inside the same cell when the mass is alone and there are no malignancies outside of the eye. Retinoblastomas are unspecialized, malignant neuroblastic growths. The child might have an odd look in the eye, and the doctor could find an irregular red reflex when doing a check-up. There may be leukocoria and eye misalignment. Inherited and in both eyes generally shows up by age one. The non-inherited type shows up by age 2.

Use enucleation for uninherited types and big lesions. Use photocoagulation on little lesion in the back. Use cold therapy for little lesions on periphery. External-beam radiation could help the tumor go away but could create problems with sarcomas in the areas that got radiation. Use chemotherapy to make the tumors smaller when needed.

Symptoms may include lessened sight, mass that extends to vitreous and is a shade of pink, separation of retina, mass in subretina that is a shade of white and vitreous seeding. Big tumors could force the lens to the front and create glaucoma, swelling and fluid in the cornea, spreading to beyond the globe which makes the eye bulge, swelling and fluid in the conjunctiva and inflammation in the inside of the eye. Some people also have blood or pus in the anterior chamber. Trilateral retinoblastoma is a case of retinoblastoma in both eyes along with a tumor in the pineal gland. Do MRI or CT and hereditary analysis. Progression may be endophytic or exophytic. Retinoblastoma can penetrate the optic nerve and go into the brain by way of subarachnoid area. The prediction is contingent upon how far along the problem is when it is identified. Finding it early and getting proper medical attention gives the person a 90% chance of survival. Sight is contingent upon measurements and region.

Medulloepithelioma, also called dictyoma – Tumor in the uncolored epithelium in the ciliary body that shows up as a mass inside the eye. It is caused by irregular growth of the retina as an embryo and creates malignancy and tumor. It usually shows up around age 5. Patient indications are redness in the eye (attributed to glaucoma or bleeding in the eye), lessened sight and lengthened lessened sight could cause eye misalignment. You may see gradually worsening tumor in ciliary body or iris that makes an irregular red reflex, random bleeding in the vitreous and glaucoma. 2/3 of people with this condition have metastatic lesions. The condition could spread into areas outside of the eye. The best medical attention is enucleation. The prediction for the future is not as good when the tumor goes through the optic nerve or into areas exterior to the eye. Watch the case carefully for spreading. Similar symptoms may indicate present at birth iris cyst, juvenile xanthogranuloma or retinoblastoma.

Dermoid cysts – In a child, it frequently is seen in the margin where the zygomatic and frontal bones meet. They are choristomas coming from ectodermal offshoots. They have an inside surface of epithelium and are filled with keratin and cholesterol. Frequently they also have hair follicles and sebaceous glands. They get stuck on the joining areas during the growth of the face. Patient indications are periobital lump that gets bigger and is commonly seen for the first time after an injury on the area. You may see a gradual growth of cystic mass located on the temporal side of the brow, big masses that can sometimes make the globe go out of position and linked body faults. An effect deep in the orbit is not usually seen in kids. Use CT when needed. Sometimes it randomly breaks causing ongoing flare-up. Cut it out and be sure to get every bit out. Do not break the lesion when cutting it out. Similar symptoms may indicate orbital encephalocele, hemangioma or dacryocystocele.

Teratomas – Germ cell tumor; congenital; created quick bulging eyeball; puts the globe in danger if not cut out. The mass is big and quickly tears down the bony orbit. The orbit gets bigger when an operation is not done. Do CT to make sure it is not going into the cranium. It is not usually malignant. With no medical attention, there may be bare keratopathy and the person may lose the eye. Drain the fluid and cut it out to save the globe. Observe for malignancy. Similar symptoms may indicate cellulitis in the orbit, rhabdomyosarcoma or retinoblastoma.

Tuberous sclerosis –Derived from Bourneville's disease; autosomal dominant due to chromosome 9. You will see nervous system tumor from astrocytes in the retina or optic nerve. There may be seizures, a range of lessened mental ability and more indications contingent upon the region. In the body there may be achromic nevi, café-au-lait places, shagreen skin, and astrocytic benign growth in the central nervous system or benign growths affecting the kidneys, bone or heart.

Juvenile xanthogranuloma – Histiocytic problem that makes the skin have lesions during babyhood and sometimes creates problems in the eye, uvea or orbit. There is quick growth of lymphocytes, plasma cells and histiocytes which are inside the skin and eyes of kids that have it. It generally arises before the first birthday (85% of cases), generally has no indications, and can randomly bleed. You may see nodes in the iris, random blood in the anterior chamber, ongoing eye inflammation, glaucoma, one eye with a different color than the other, and very uncommon instances of affect in the optic nerve. The body may have yellow, pimply lesions on the skin. Do a tissue sample study to verify identification of the condition. The condition gets better on its own by the beginning teenage years. Cutting it out is not recommended since it is likely to bleed. Corticosteroids can be used and may cause remission. Radiation may be utilized if steroids are not working. Similar symptoms may indicate retinoblastoma, medulloepithelioma, leukemic infiltration or neuroblastoma.

Phakomatoses

Angiomatosis retinae – Name derived from von Hippel-Lindau disease; autosomal dominant from chromosome 3. You may see capillary hemangiomas in the retina and linked bleeding and exudates. The body may have benign tumors in the cerebellum, malignant tumor of the renal cells, pheochromocytomas, cyst in the pancreas, liver or epididymis. Progression is contingent upon location and is more commonly seen in fully-grown people.

Ataxia-telangiectasia – Name derived from Louis-Bar syndrome; autosomal recessive from chromosome 11. You may see enlarged blood vessels near the surface of the conjunctiva and lack of ability of the eyeball to move voluntarily. In the body, there may be blood vessels near the surface of the skin and underdeveloped thymus. Ataxia in the cerebellum gets worse from age 2. The patient may have respiratory tract infections and lessened mental ability along with problems with moving the eyeball.

Racemose angioma – Name derived from Wyburn-Mason syndrome; there is not a clear hereditary design, irregular blood vessel development in the retina, and the body may have irregular blood vessel and artery development in the cranium. The patient will have lessened mental ability and more neurological problems (contingent upon region).

Neurofibromatosis type I – Name derived from von Recklinghausen's disease; autosomal dominant from chromosome 17. This is the most frequently seen phakomatosis out of 4000 people who have it. You may see optic nerve glioma, lisch protuberances, glaucoma on the same side as a tumor in a nerve on the lid, a tumor in a nerve on the conjunctiva, bigger corneal nerves, pulsatile bulging of the eyeball that comes from irregularities on the sphenoid. You may see café-au-lait patches, tumors coming from nerves, armpit and groin freckling, underdevelopment of the sphenoid, glioma or tumor in the adrenal gland. The indications are contingent upon the kind and region of the problem. The person may have seizures and a range of lessened mental ability.

Encephalofacial angiomatosis – Name derived from Sturge-Weber syndrome; hemangioma in the choroid, glaucoma that affects the lid or conjunctiva on the same side. The person might also have hemangioma on the face, meninges or in the central nervous system. The birthmark will be there when the child is born. There may be problems with seizures, a range of lessened mental ability and more indications (contingent upon region).

Neurofibromatosis type 2 – Autosomal dominant from chromosome 22; cataracts in the posterior subcapsular area, optic nerve glioma and tumor in the meninges. In the body, there may be acoustic tumor in the nerve cells on both sides, central nervous system glioma, tumor in the meninges or tumor in the adrenal gland. The patient may experience lessened ability to hear, dizziness, seizure or a range of lessened mental ability.

Pierre-Robin sequence – Marked with cleft palate, linked to underdeveloped mandible. You may see a lot of nearsightedness, separation in the retina, small eyes, cataract and glaucoma. Similar symptoms may indicate Stickler syndrome.

Craniofacial Malformations

Goldenhar syndrome (oculoauricular dysostosis) – Linked to the eyeball dermoid in the cornea or conjunctiva; linked to preauricular parts. The irregularity is due to unusual differentiation in the mesoderm that derives from the first branchial arch. This condition is random. You may see dermoid or lipodermoid on the cornea or conjunctiva, small eyes, and coloboma on the lid (generally top lid). In the body, there may be an affect in the preauricular parts or passages, irregularities in the vertebrae, present at birth heart disease and irregularities in the central nervous system. Big colobomas can cause bare keratopathy. Dermoid in the cornea could cause a lot of astigmatism and lazy eye because of the block or provoked lazy eye with noteworthy different refractive powers in each eye. Medical attention includes plastic surgery to mend coloboma on lids, management for bare keratopathy, and cutting out dermoid problems. Similar symptoms may indicate Treacher Collins syndrome.

Waardenburg syndrome – One iris a different color from the other, loss of hearing, white lock of hair on the forehead, widely spaced eyes and inside corners of the eyes set far apart. Similar symptoms may indicate present at birth Horner syndrome.

Craniosynostosis syndromes – Autosomal dominant; early shutting of sutures in the cranium, generally together with another form of irregular growth. It commonly causes an orbit that is not deep, bulging eye and more. The patient may have underdeveloped upper jaw bone, projection of bottom jaw and shallow orbit including eyes that look to be bulging. You may find swelling around the optic nerve due to pressure on the nerve or in the cranium, bare cornea, eye misalignment, V-design eye misalignment due to irregular orbit development. The body may have Crouzon's disease, Apert syndrome or Pfeiffer syndrome. Carefully observed the child for raised IOP and lesions that occur due to ongoing pressure on the optic nerve. There is a chance of exposure keratopathy. Use moisturizers or shielding moisture chambers.

Fetal alcohol syndrome – Abnormal embryo development due to contact with alcohol during the first trimester. The baby may be born early and have intrauterine slowed development. You may see ptosis in both eyes with smaller measurement of lids, droopy lids, wide-set eye openings, underdevelopment of optic nerve, abnormal development of anterior segment or eye misalignment. The child may have developmental delay, present at birth heart disease and irregular face features including a lack of philtrum and wide top lip. There is no medical attention. Similar symptoms may indicate dilantin embyopathy or cocaine embryopathy.

Albinism

Albinism is present at birth problem in the melanin system which causes lessened color in the skin alone, skin and eyes, or eyes alone.

- Oculocutaneous albinism – autosomal recessive; could be total or patieal and have a range of sign. The patient may have white hair, pink skin, light sensitivity and quick and involuntary eye movements.
- Ocular albinism – autosomal recessive of X-associated; may have light sensitivity, quick and involuntary eye movements and light coloration of skin.

You may find nystagmus, problems with the iris transillumination, hypoplasia in the fovea, lessened pigment epithelium in the retina, lessened sight, irregular sight corridors including lessened amount of uncrossed fibers on the chiasm and irregular stacking of lateral geniculate nucleus. As the pigment is lessened, the vision is lessened and the patient experiences more indications. There may be Chediak-Higashi syndrome, a very uncommon form of oculocutaneous albinism with irregular retinuloendothelial system and reappearing infections, lessened mental ability, lymphadenopathy, hepatosplenomegaly and giant irregular cytoplasmic granules inside white blood cells. There may be Hermansky-Pudlak syndrome (form of oculocutaneous albinism linked to platelet fault and effortless bruising). Use a hair bulb assessment to see if tyrosinase was substituted with hereditary study. The problems in the eyes will not alter as time goes by. Pigmentation will not be added to. Nystagmus commonly lessens. Use tinted lenses to handle light sensitivity. Tinted contacts may be used. The patient should see a low-vision specialist in the early years to make proper arrangements for instruction.

Crytherapy and Laser Photocoagulation

Cryotherapy – Used for an acute instance of ROP; higher chance of cardiopulmonary problems with this treatment than with photocoagulation. Enlarge the pupils and put in lid speculum. Do cryotherapy on the whole peripheral avascular zone with a manually held cryo-pencil. Look at the periphery of the retina while handling the cryo-pencil to depress the sclera. What you want is a white freeze place for 1-2 seconds. Lesions are positioned next to the area.

Laser photocoagulation – Some accounts say that this treatment gives 90% chance of threshold retinopathy of prematurity getting better. When it does get better, you will see a lessening of plus disease within one week, but there might not very much difference in the fibrovascular growth outside the retina at that point (but it should begin to lessen by the second week). For the 10% of patients who do not respond to this treatment, additional medical attention will be needed.

Treating Retinopathy

When a second treatment for retinopathy of prematurity should be done – Do laser photocoagulation again if the problem actually gets worse in the first week, the disease is unrelenting, there are places where the laser did not handle the problem (skip lesions) or lesions that are far apart when two weeks have gone by. Use extra medical attention on places that did not get handled the first time instead of going back over places that the laser handled before. Extra cryotherapy may be used for skip areas as well when the first time was not enough.

Medical attention needed for stages 4A, 4B and 5 – Stage 4A that is worsening with time and stage 4B are treated utilizing an operation for scleral buckling. This gives the person a 60% chance of retinal reattachment. There is a 35% chance of the baby who has an attached retina of attaining useful sight. Surgical removal of the vitreous can be utilized in stage 5, but the chances of a good outcome are not very bad.

Late problems -- Later problems are nearsightedness, pigmentation in the retina, movement of the retina, deterioration of the retina and vitreous in a lattice pattern, separation of the retina and angle closure glaucoma. There may also be lazy eye and eye misalignment. Anyone that has later stages of ROP should get ongoing check-ups with a retina specialist and pediatric ophthalmologist.

Down Syndrome

Down syndrome is trisomy in chromosome 21 and is frequently seen in babies with moms that are older than 35. This is marked with big tongue, face hypoplasia, epicanthal folds, short and webbed neck, short fingers, palmar crease, present at birth heart disease including endocardial cushion faults and irregularities in the gastrointestinal region. In the eye you may see blepharitis due to slack lids, frequently the person will have refractive problems such as hyperopia, nearsightedness, astigmatism or keratoconus, nystagmus or strabismus. In young adults, snowflake cataracts arise. Present at birth infantile cataracts are common. There may be Brushfield spots. Check the chromosome to verify the condition.

Aicardi Syndrome

Aicardi syndrome is marked with optic nerve underdevelopment linked to transparent cavity in the retina. In a male child, it is fatal; therefore you will only see female children with this condition. The patient indications are seizures in the early years, spasms in the infant and lessened mental ability. Use an MRI to see marks of gray matter irregularities and ectopic gray matter will be there as well. There will be no corpus callosum. The seizures are very hard to manage but should get medical attention.

Nystagmus

Latent nystagmus – Generally seen in someone that has present at birth cross-eye; this nystagmus happens if either one of the eyes is obscured. There may be dissociated vertical deviation. The jerk movement happens towards the eye that is not obscured. The problem stays the same over the years and is not linked to any other central nervous system problem.

Confusion – Unlike images are seen on equivalent retinal images so that one overlies the other.

Congenital nystagmus – In both eyes, big nystagmus that goes across and is commonly depicted as wandering motion of the eye. It is seen in people that have bad sight in both eyes due to an irregular optic nerve. It is not related to cortical blindness. Once it arises, it generally cannot be made better. The problem comes up by the time the baby is 3 months old. Horizontal nystagmus is in both upgaze and downgaze. There will be head bobbing, opposite response in the pupil (get smaller in dark, bigger in light), turn head to diminish problem, lack of problem when asleep, and lack of involuntary eye movements or feeling of moving. The optokinetic nystagmus reaction is reversed.

Diplopia – The exact images are seen on different retinal regions so that the person gets double vision. It can be in one or both eyes.

Spasmus nutans – Fast back-and-forth movement of the eyes; not harmful; linked to bobbing head and torticollis. It generally starts from 3 to 18 months and gets better by age 3 or 4. The nystagmus has little amplitude but a fast rate of speed. It is generally in both eyes but some people have it in only one, in an unbalanced way or a range of other ways. With the bobbing head, the nystagmus is not as much. Use MRI to make sure there is no central nervous system tumor.

Yoke Muscles

Yoke muscles are two muscles working together to make the eye go in the direction of gaze that the person wants. The ways the yoke muscles work together are as follows:

- Movement to the right – right lateral rectus to left medial rectus
- Movement to the top and right – right superior rectus to left inferior oblique
- Movement to the top and left – left superior rectus to right inferior oblique
- Movement to the left – left lateral rectus to right medial rectus
- Movement to the bottom and left – left inferior rectus to right superior oblique
- Movement to the bottom and right – right inferior rectus to left superior oblique

Extraocular Muscles

The extraocular muscles, measurements and the movements of each starting at the main position:

- Medial rectus – 37.7mm long; 3.0mm tendon length; 5.7mm from the place where it goes in to the limbus; main position adduction
- Inferior rectus – 37.0mm long; 4.7mm tendon length; 6.7mm from the place where it goes in to the limbus; main position depression, secondary position excycloduction; tertiary position adduction
- Lateral rectus – 36.3mm long; 7.2mm tendon length; 7.0 mm from the place where it goes in to the limbus; main position abduction
- Superior rectus – 37.0mm long; 4.0mm tendon length; 8.0 mm from the place where it goes in to the limbus; main position elevation; secondary position incycloduction; tertiary position adduction
- Inferior oblique – 37.0mm long; 1.5mm tendon length; 17.5 – 20.0 mm from the place where it goes in to the limbus; main position excycloduction; secondary position elevation; tertiary position abduction
- Superior oblique – 59.5mm long; 19.5mm tendon length; 14.0 – 18.0 mm from the place where it goes in to the limbus; main position incycloduction; secondary position depression; tertiary position abduction

Hering's and Sherington's Laws

Hering's law of equal innervation – Equivalent and happening at the same time nerve stimulation streams to synergistic muscles that have to do with the wanted direction of gaze. This means that if the person wants to see something to the left, equivalent innervation prompt will occur in the right medial rectus and left lateral rectus.

Sherington's law – More constriction of a muscle outside but near the eye goes along with lessened contractile motion in the opponent of that eye. For instance, when looking to the left gaze, the left lateral rectus is the agonist. It is provoked into constriction. The left medial rectus is the opponent and is repressed.

Fusion and Rivalry

Sensory fusion – Working together of sight exitations, beginning at equivalent retinal images and coming together to form one image alone in sight.

Motor fusion – The capacity to line up the eyes to keep sensory fusion in working order.

Retinal rivalry – Occurs if different images are demonstrated to the equivalent regions of the retina; provokes fusion.

Suppression, ARC and Stereopsis

Suppression – Sensory variation of double vision which stops images in an eye from getting to the person's consciousness.

Anomalous retinal correspondence (ARC) – Sensory variation that happens for people who have strabismus so that each fovea is going it its own deviating visual way.

Harmonious ARC – Occurs if the angle of the abnormality is equivalent to the deviation of the strabismus

Unharmonious ARC – Occurs if the angle of the irregularity is less than the angle in strabismus

Stereopsis – Comparative arrangement of images in depth that happens when the horizontal dissimilar images in the retina are provoked at random. It is measured in seconds of arc. A normal one would have 15 – 30 seconds of arc.

Ambyopia

Amblyopia can occur in one or both eyes; lessened vision due to form vision deficiency or irregular ability of the two eyes to work together with no natural reason found during evaluation (but may be fixed with medical attention if the person is young). The forms include:

- Visual deprivation – Present at birth cataract, cloudiness in the cornea, bleeding in the vitreous; worst type and hardest to handle.
- Strabismic - Seen more frequently with cross-eye; happens along with suppression
- Anisometropic – Unbalanced refractive problems; best in terms of being able to handle it with medical attention

Medical attention choices include occlusion treatment, patching for some or all of the time and penalization with atropine in the good eye to make the image fuzzy when viewing it from a close distance. A person who is under the age of 5 can get occlusion lazy eye (a risk with patching all the time). The use of occlusion can make the lazy eye better for a person who has the anisometropic form if done before the person is 13. Occlusion treatment for some of the time gives more binocular ability but does not work as quickly to correct lazy eye.

Strabismus

When checking for strabismus, find out what issues occurred prior to birth such as any illness in the mother, smoking, drug or alcohol issues or diabetes. Find out any issues that occurred during the baby's birth including how the baby was born, anoxic/hypoxic occurrences, gestational age at birth, birth weight, bleeding in the ventricular areas, and how long the hospital stay lasted.

Find out when the problem began. Ask how old the patient was, whether there was linked injury, sickness, how often it happens, pattern, reverting symptoms, provoking elements such as the sun, sickness or exhaustion as well as any elements that make it get better, and linked indications such as head pain, light sensitivity or neurological irregularities. Find out about prior sicknesses, family accounts of the same problem and go over the systems. Ask about weight fluctuation, how quickly the person gets tired, high blood pressure, diabetes, head pain or neurological indications. Check strabismus and sensorimotor.

Checking for Strabismus:

Cover evaluation for heterotropia (one eye does not line up with target) - block the eye that can fixate and see the reaction from the other eye. If it moves to the outside, this is a sign of cross-eye, but inside is a sign of wall-eye. Moving down is hypertropia, but moving up is hypotropia. Do it on both eyes. It is useful to quickly know the tropia. The con is that there must be fixation and it cannot find little amounts of tropia or phoria.

Cover/uncover assessment for heterophoria – this condition is one where fusion is sustained with binocular sight. If one eye is blocked, the phoria may be seen with the difference in the covered eye. But the block on one eye. Take it off and look at that eye. The action in that eye is a sign that there is phoria. It is good because it quickly finds phoria, but the con is that there must be fixation and it cannot find little irregularities.

Assessments to measure amount of strabismus deviation include Hirschberg test, Krimsky test, prism cover test, Maddox rod test for heterophoria, double Maddox rod test for cyclodeviation and

3-step test for cyclovertical palsy. Stereopsis tests include: titmus stereo Polaroid test and random dot stereogram.

Estropia

Congenital (infantile) esotropia – Cross-eye that shows up prior to the time the baby is 6 months old. It is unclear what the causes is, but may be a main fault in the sensory fusion system or main fault in motor fusion. The patient experiences a big difference that is generally more than 45 prism diopters between the two eyes and alternating fixation/cross-fixation. There is frequently someone else in the family that has had strabismus. You may find it with a big angle, interchanging fixation, cross-fixation (which may look like 6th-nerve palsy in both eyes), lazy eye in rare instances, refractive problem that is +2.00 sphere or under. As time goes by there may be inferior oblique overworking, dissociated vertical deviation (DVD) or dormant nystagmus.

With no medical attention the person will have good sight including free interchanging fixation, lack of ability of two eyes to work together to see, DVD and you will frequently see oblique overwork. Someone with medical attention can get the eyes to work together in the periphery, gross stereopsis may arise, DVD, dormant nystagmus and oblique overwork are frequently seen. Treat lazy eye by using occlusion treatment, attempt the use of glasses if refraction is +1.50 sphere or higher, and the person will generally need an operation. When to do the operation is debatable since some think an earlier operation gets greater amount of sensory fusion but some think it only needs to be by age 2. The majority use surgery from ages 9 – 16 months. The operation is bimedial recession. If the irregularity is more than 45 prism diopters, do this surgery together with lateral rectus resection. When the oblique is overworking it will have to be weakened. Use botulinum toxin to weaken the medial rectus.

Check the person after surgery to see if lazy eye or accommodative cross-eye comes up. 30% - 40% of kids require another operation later in the lifespan. For the next 6 years afterwards, check the person twice a year to see if lazy eye arises or a reappearance of strabismus. Similar symptoms may indicate an early beginning to accommodative cross-eye, nystagmus obstruction syndrome, Duane syndrome, Moebius syndrome, abducens palsy in both eyes or sensory cross-eye.

Accommodative esotropia – Obtained form of esotropia that arises from 18 to 36 months and is caused by too much accommodation in a person that that has longsightedness. There is a synkinetic association for accommodation and convergence. A number of the patients have eyes that will accommodate to make the image clear. This causes convergence and cross-eye. A number of these patients also get a lot of accommodative convergence-to-accommodation (AC/A) proportion. This causes the eye to turn in towards the nose more when focusing on something close up.

The patient may experience eyes that cross (which may be sporadic in the beginning), an irregularity that commonly begins during near fixation and worsens to happen during distance, worse symptoms if the person is sick or tired, and double vision prior to the suppression and lazy eye arising. Although it generally begins from 18 to 36 months, it may happen anywhere from 6 months to age 7. It is common for the child to have others in the family with eye misalignment. You may find cross-eye that is 20-40 prism diopters, longsightedness, a lot of AC/A, lazy eye, bad stereopsis when the problem has been going on for a long time (but depth perception could also be fine when the problem is not constant and there is good medical attention), and some have a V design. To assess, it is vital to do cycloplegic refraction. Gauge AC/A, gauge deviation with an accommodative target for both far and close in the 9 gaze positions, and do prism adaptation evaluation.

Accommodative convergence-to-accommodation (AC/A) ratio – There are two techniques:

1. Heterophoria technique – Gauge the difference for far and near. When it is more than 10 prism diopters, the person has a big AC/A ratio.
2. Gradient technique (chosen more often) – Determine the fixed place for far or near, put +3.0 sphere in front of the person and gauge the difference again. The formula for finding the ratio is:

$$\frac{AC}{A} = \frac{deviation\ with\ lens - deviation\ with\ no\ lens}{Lens\ power}$$

Note: an AC/A ratio that is from 3 – 5 is considered normal.

With no medical attention, lazy eye arises and gets to a point where it cannot be fixed by the time the child is 6 years old and stereopsis will be gone. If the child has medical attention the sight is fixable and regular stereopsis may be kept. Longsightedness gets worse as time goes by and a number of kids might be able to stop using glasses by the time they are 10.

Ocular treatment includes total amount of hyperopia refraction. A lot of AC/A means bifocals will be needed. The bifocals will need +2.50 sphere and executive design segment to split the pupil. Glasses should be used all the time; sometimes they handle the problem totally. When the person gets older the refractive problem lessens and many times the glasses may be tapered off around age 10-12. Pharmacologic attention includes anticholinesterase drops to start accommodation on the region by taking away the fuzziness and provoking accommodation in the middle along with convergence. This works especially well to lessen AC/A ratio, but since there are consequences of using the medicine glasses should be tried first. Anticholinesterase medications include phospholine iodide 0.06% (may cause cyst creation in iris, ongoing apnea when general anesthesia is needed, provoked nearsightedness and separation in the retina), pilocarpine 1% (may cause nearsightedness or retinal separation, or diisopropyl phosphorofluoridate 0.025% ointment (may cause same problems as phospholine iodide and is effortlessly hydrolyzed when it touches water).

An operation is only done when the patient has partially accommodative esotropia and glasses to not totally get the eyes in balance or if the patient will not wear the glasses. When someone has the operation that could have had good results from glasses there will be the consequence of successive outward deviation in a few years when the longsightedness lessens. If the patient had partially accommodative cross-eye then the surgery done needs to only be for the left over difference that cannot be fixed with glasses. Use the prism adaptation assessment to find out how much needs to be righted. Lazy eye has to be checked and tended to. Check binocularity each time the person comes in. When the eyes are balanced with glasses and lazy eye is fixed, check back every 4-6 months. Do cycloplegic refraction each year. Taper off the use of glasses from 8 to 11 years of age. Similar symptoms may indicate infantile cross-eye, sixth-nerve palsy or Duane syndrome.

Exodeviation

Exodeviation is an unbalanced lining up of sight axes; dormant with fusion (exophoria) or could come and go (intermittent wall-eye), or may always be there (constant wall-eye). Causes include mechanical elements, craniofacial problems, disproportion in convergent/divergence, or if the sight is bad it may be sensory wall-eye. The patient may experience more indications when tired or looking at something far away, double vision sometimes, asthenopia, narrowing of eyes and light sensitivity. This condition is frequently in kids more than 2 years old. An intermittent case can worsen to be there all the time. Lazy eye is not usually seen, but suppression arises easily. Under examination, you may find a number of indications that are contingent upon the form of wall-eye that the patient has. These include basic wall-eye, divergence excess wall-eye, stimulated divergence excess or convergence insufficiency. If the child has present at birth wall-eye along with neurological irregularities a pediatric neurological assessment is required. There may be craniofacial problems such as Crouzon's disease or Apert syndrome. V-design may be the case.

Use prolonged occlusion evaluation by blocking an eye for 30-45 minutes to unlink the eyes maximally and temporarily stop fusion. It lets you get the distance of the most deviation. Get measurements for both far and near. Use +3.00 sphere assessments to temporarily stop accommodation. As time goes by, outward turning could create eye strain, worsen to discontinuous deviation, or intermittent exodeviation could begin by only affecting far fixation but worsen to affect near and lessen stereo acuity.

Medical attention for lessened convergence includes convergence exercises. If convergence is fine, think about base-in prism to help patient. For wall-eye that comes and goes, handle lazy eye and refractive problems. If the child is under 3 years old, try occlusion for some of the time that he is awake. Use minus lenses that are –1.50 to –3.00D sphere to provoke accommodation which will help wall-eye. Problems with convergence may be helped with eye exercises. Base-in prisms are used when another treatment (excepting an operation) will not handle the problem.

Operations are only for cases that come and go and the problem is getting bigger and faster or wall-eye all the time. Divergence excess wall-eye is handled with two-sided lateral rectus recessions. Wall-eye that is present all the time and sensory wall-eye need recession or resection methods. Problems with convergence are handled with two-sided medial resection.

30% of people that have had surgery get exodeviation that comes back again. This happens more often when the person has sensory wall-eye. Similar symptoms may indicate third-nerve paresis or Duane syndrome type II adduction insufficiency.

Dissociated vertical deviation (DVD), also called divergent vertical deviation, alternating sursumduction, and disassociative hypertropia – one eye gradually moves up and out along with excyclotorsion action. It happens on its own or if that eye is blocked. When the block is taken off, the eye depresses, intorsion occurs, and it adducts to the place it was prior to block. The other eye will not move (breach of Hering's law) making this problem different from real hypertropia.

Vertical Deviation

The reason for the problem is not known, but some people think it has to do with a supranuclear problem, too much activity in the superior rectus muscle, and universally more tone in the extraocular muscles. The patient will not have double vision because of suppression. One eye moves up when the child is tired or distracted. The person will have prior infantile cross-eye or another type of eye misalignment that began as a baby. You may see raising, abduction and extorsion when the eye is blocked. It is mostly in both eyes but can be unbalanced and a times also comes with inferior oblique overwork. When looking to the opposite direction the DVD gets worse. Look at Bielschowsky's phenomenon to assess. This is in regards to the propensity for the raised eye to come down if light in the fixing eye is lessened. It happens if the eye coming down is under a block.

Generally this is a worsening-with-time problem. Medical attention is needed if the problem changes the way the person looks. Treat any refractive problems because fuzzy sight makes DVD worse. When the problem is unbalanced, making the uninfluenced eye fuzzy on purpose can help. It may go along with putting too much plus in the fixating eye to manage DVD in the other eye. An operation is probably needed for DVD in both eyes. In both eyes, superior rectus recession needs the hang-back method. Posterior fixation sutures can be put in for superior rectus recession. Anteriorization for inferior obliques may be used with DVD that includes too much work from the inferior oblique. Similar symptoms may indicate too much work from inferior oblique, but that gives a V-design; DVD does not do A or V designs. Eye torsion will always be with DVD and never in inferior oblique overwork. DVD the speed of elevation is slow but inferior oblique overaction is quick. 40% have both DVD and inferior oblique overaction.

Double Elevator Palsy

Double elevator palsy is when one cannot raise an eye. Three things may cause this condition:

1. Inferior rectus restriction including positive forced duction assessment and normal saccade speed in the superior rectus muscle.
2. Elevator muscle is not strong enough; identified with no limit on forced duction assessment and lessened force creation of elevators including lessened saccadic speed for upgaze of that eye.
3. The person may have both of the above at the same time.

The patient may experience no ability to raise the eye and irregular head position can be mistaken for fusion. Pseudoptosis occurs in a case where the hypotropic depressed eye can fixate which makes the seeming ptosis get better. That is something that generally arises for a young person. You may find hypotropia on the main position, lack of ability to raise the eye and pseudoptosis. It generally needs an operation. Do forced duction assessment during at the same time as the operation. Similar symptoms may indicate Brown syndrome or blowout fracture.

When there is thyroid eye disease, the inferior rectus muscle frequently is influenced and the person can also get limiting eye misalignment. Fourth-nerve palsy also includes the positive head angle assessment outcome that does not aid in identifying double elevator palsy.

Superior Oblique Palsy

Superior oblique palsy can be present at birth or caused by an injury; may include hypertropis on that eye. The person will frequently have an irregular head tilt in the direction opposite from the ineffective muscle. People who have had it from birth do not usually have double vision. The irregular head tilt is more frequently seen in an obtained condition. The cause from birth is usually no known, although it could occur following a virus. An obtained case is commonly caused by hurting the head in some way. The patient may experience hyper- or hypotropia, angled head, unbalanced face and double vision with torsion.

When looking at the fundus with a circuitous ophthalmoscope you may see objective cycloextorsion. There may be a V-design of cross-eye when the person has fourth-nerve palsy on both sides. Look for excyclotorsion with a double Maddox rod; it might be more than 8° if the person has two-sided superior oblique palsy. When looking for the difference between a case that is present at birth and a case that was obtained later, look at the following:

- Present at birth – problem will have been there for years with big vertical fusion amplitude and an unbalanced face. Look at pictures from the person's lifespan for signs. The problem is commonly managed by angling the head.
- Obtained later – double vision, images seem angled, may or may not have angled head and/or unbalanced face, but the vertical fusion amplitude is fine. The person might get inflexible double vision, torsional double vision and lose fusion as time goes by.

Some people get double vision around 15-35 years old due to deviation alterations.

To assess, use Park's 3-step assessment and double Maddox rod test. When the hypertropia is small than 15 prism diopters the problem may be managed by deteriorating the inferior oblique on the same side. When it is more, think about doing an operation for more vertical muscle. The inferior rectus muscle on the other side may be pushed back with a variable suture process. When the superior rectus on the other side is tight during forced duction assessment, push that muscle back. Be careful when doing surgery on these muscles since the outcome could be too much adjustment. Use sutures that can be altered with this condition. If the person has noteworthy underwork in the superior oblique muscle, utilize a tuck for the superior oblique tendon. It can have an outcome of eye misalignment and Brown syndrome caused by medical attention. Two-sided superior oblique palsy needs a process to diminish the inferior oblique. When the instance is obtained superior oblique paresis including torsion, use Harade-Ito process. Similar symptoms may indicate dissociated vertical divergence, too much work from the inferior oblique or skew divergence.

Brown Syndrome

Brown syndrome is a constricting type of eye misalignment; restriction on how the eye is raised during adduction. It is a problem with the superior oblique tendon and trochlea that make the tissue denser than normal in the region inside and surrounding the trochlea. This stops the tendon from moving smoothly. It can be present at birth or obtained later. The patient may have double vision when looking in the main position and use a chin-up head tilt to make up for the problem during abduction. It might hurt around the trochlea area and there can be an irregular feeling or snap around that area at the time of raising/adducting the eye. Similar symptoms may indicate inferior oblique palsy, present at birth formation of fibrous tissue, double elevator palsy, blowout fracture, thyroid myopathy or adherence problem.

Constriction or total lack of raising the eye during adduction, constriction of palpebral fissure during adduction, a lack of overwork from the superior oblique on the same side, wall-eye when looking up in a V-design, chin-up head tilt in order to aid sight and common instances of orthotropia when looking in the main position. There might be downshoot on that eye during adduction. The forced duction assessment will be positive every time if the person has this condition. The problem may be linked to injury, a tumor that has spread into the orbit, ethmoid sinus operation, Marfan syndrome, rheumatoid arthritis, acromegaly, a tooth being taken out, an operation for retinal separation or an operation for glaucoma seton. Use the Guyton provoking traction assessment. If the problem is obtained, an imaging study of the orbit may be needed.

With Brown syndrome it is important to manage the main cause. Use regional insertion of triamcinolone or methylprednisolone on the trochlea if there is flare-up (temporary; may need more than one). Some people do not need medical attention. Noteworthy hypotropia and noteworthy chin-up angle may require deterioration method on the superior oblique muscle. Do tenotomy on the superior oblique tendon, but it could have an outcome of paralyzing the superior oblique and the inferior oblique would then have to be weakened to handle the following hypertropia. All of this can be done in one surgery. Utilizing silicone tendon expander is encouraged to get the tendon to loosen up with no resulting paresis on the superior oblique muscle.

A and V Patterns

A and V patterns are common muscle problems, especially with strabismus that has been there for a long time; esotropia or wall-eye that alters in degree from up to downgaze.

Horizontal eye misalignment; horizontal alteration is different in amount for upgaze and downgaze. Clinically noteworthy A design has up-and-down incomitant horizontal strabismus with 10 prism diopters and more coming together when looking up. Clinically noteworthy V design has up-and-down incomitant eye misalignment with 15 prism diopters including more coming together when looking down.

There may be oblique muscle problems. Too much work from the inferior oblique is linked to V-design; too much superior oblique is linked to A. There may be horizontal muscle problems. Too much work from medial rectus is linked to V during downgaze and is frequently linked to two-sided lateral recti muscles being not strong enough. The face may have problems. A person with mongoloid elements can get A-design cross-eye and V-design wall-eyes. Someone with no mongoloid features has the opposite: A-design wall-eye and V-design cross-eye. There can be slight two-sided 6th nerve paresis. Neurological problems that are linked to A-design are hydrocephalus, Arnold-Chiari development problems and posterior fossa disease. You may find V-design wall-eye with Brown syndrome. A-design wall-eye is linked to too much work in the superior obliques. Make sure there are no neurological problems when the A or V pattern is noteworthy.

If horizontal eye misalignment goes on a long time, vertical eye misalignment can arise. Gauge the difference from up to downgaze and be sure that the target is at the same place for both (very important). When there is not an oblique muscle problem, crumple the design by moving the horizontal muscles towards the location of the wanted weakness or from the location that needs the most amplification. For instance, if there is V-design cross-eye, manage it by pushing back the medial recti muscles and moving them 1 tendon width down. If managing A-design cross-eye with the method of making the superior oblique muscle less strong, make to keep away from stimulation or torsion. Think about doing posterior subtotal 7/8ths tenotomy instead. The use of making the inferior oblique muscles less strong on both sides fixes 15-25 prism diopters of V. Two-sided superior oblique tenotomy can fix 45 prism diopters for A and have an outcome of 45 prism diopters for the downgaze esoshift.

Duane Retraction Syndrome

Duane retractioni syndrome is generally restricted ability to abduct in an eye along with the eye sinking into the socket during the time that the movement is tried. With electromyography it has been shown that there is lessened work from the lateral rectus when abduction is tried using contradictory use of nerves from the lateral rectus in adduction. The patient may have to turn the face to keep fusion and make double vision go away. There may be up- or downshoots when adduction is tried. It may run in the family as an autosomal dominant condition, and 30% - 50% also have another form of present at birth irregularity. 15% have it in both eyes. You may see the globe retract during adduction, the lid shut a little bit along with enophthalmos during adduction, no movement or reduced work during convergence on that eye, lazy eye and a bit of cross-eye. Tightening the horizontal recti at the same time has an outcome of retraction in the globe when adduction is happening.

Duane retraction syndrome includes three forms:

- Type I – lessened abduction
- Type II – lessened adduction
- Type III – lessening of both

In 16%, the person also has sensorineural inability to hear. Some patients also have Goldenhar syndrome. As it progresses, the person might have to turn the head even more to balance the eyes and stop double vision from occurring. Watch the case at first. If the problem is causing noteworthy turning of the head, an operation may be done to recess the medial rectus muscle on the same side. Moving the vertical recti to the side rectus may be done to heighten the abduction when there is a lot of cross-eye and the person has to turn his head a lot. Use Faden suture to handle any up- or downshoot. Similar symptoms may indicate 6th nerve palsy, blowout fracture including snare of the medial rectus or double vision along with lessened jerky speed during abduction.

Moebius Syndrome

Moebius syndrome includes a number of cranial nerve palsies and influences nerves VI and VII; linked to having underdeveloped tongue. It is thought to be present at birth due to harm done during week four or five of development. It also may be due to a blood vessel problem that caused reduced blood flow or fluid and swelling in the bulbar nerves. The person may experience a flat facial appearance, limited ability to move the eyes back and forth, droopy eyelid, problems with eating (due to the tongue), and trouble shutting the lid all the way. You will frequently see strabismic lazy eye, bad ability to fuse, bare keratopathy (due to lagophthalmos), horizontal gaze palsy and a range of form of cross-eye. Handle the strabismic lazy eye utilizing a block treatment, manage the problems shutting the lid with moisturizers, and recessions may be used.

Congenital Fibrosis Syndrome

Congenital fibrosis syndrome is lessened ability to move eye from the influenced muscle. Do forced duction assessment. It may be random or autosomal dominant. The muscles outside of (but near) the eye have primary fibrosis. The muscles have irregular denervation and as a result of that there are fibrotic alterations. The patient may experience no capability to move eyes, marked chin-up head tilt along with ptosis, and eyes that are stuck looking down and cross-eye. Every extraocular muscle is affected along with linked droopy lid. If the condition only affects inferior rectus muscle it may look like double elevator palsy. Strabismus fixus affects the horizontal recti and includes significant cross-eye. When the forced duction assessment comes out negatively, think about myasthenia gravis. Lazy eye is linked to this condition. The person may need surgery to help the irregular angle of the head. Recessing the constricted muscles has to be big with the hang-back method. Manage ptosis utilizing brow suspension. Similar symptoms may indicate double elevatory palsy, Brown syndrome or myasthenia gravis.

Thyroid Eye Disease

Thyroid eye disease is most frequently seen form of obtained double vision for a fully grown person; lymphocytic penetration into the muscles around the eye that causes swelling and fluid, flare-up and fibrosis in those muscles and eye misalignment as a secondary problem. It is an autoimmune condition where the antibodies go in opposition to the shared thyroid-orbital antigens and causes too much creation of flare-up mediators. The patient may experience conjunctiva swelling or injection in the conjunctiva, swelling and fluid in the lid, bulging eyeball, inability to shut lid and bare keratopathy, double vision and lessened sight due to optic nerve pressure. It is more frequently found in females and more frequently seen from age 20-40. Werner categorized this condition. The double vision is worse when looking up; inferior rectus muscle is affected most often, medial rectus affected second most often, and lateral rectus muscles affected third most often.

You will see constriction of action in the up direction and forced duction will be positive. There is heightened IOP when looking up which is a sign of restrictive eye misalignment. The person may also have hyper- or hypothyroidism and can be euthyroid. Do a lab test on the thyroid and think about doing an imaging study on the optic nerve. Check vision when the optic nerve may be affected. Do CT or MRI to look at the muscles around the eye (which will be bigger than normal). The tendon will not be bigger. The case may be acute or ongoing. When acute, there is flare-up penetration in the muscles around the eye. The eye misalignment can be temporary or may range. After flare-up stage, there may be a fibrotic phase when eye misalignment can become unfixable.

For acute thyroid disease, use corticosteroids in the body (which will help the eye misalignment). The person has to have a normal thyroid gland 3. Handle pressure on optic nerve with corticosteroids, radiation treatment or decompression of orbit. An operation for strabismus needs to be postponed until pressure on optic nerve is handled. If the strabismus has small angle, handle double vision with prism glasses. If acute, use Botulinum injection. If the condition is fibrotic, wait 4-6 months to do operation so that the difference will be known for sure. Handle hypotropia with recessing the inferior rectus muscle. Use adjustable suture and allow a bit of undercorrection. An overcorrection that occurs later is frequently seen in this type of condition. Fix cross-eye with recession of inferior rectus muscle. When the medial rectus muscle is constricted during forced duction, think about recessing it with adjustable sutures. If there is wall-eye after the surgery, check for myasthenia gravis (which arises in 70% of people who have Grave's disease).

Cryotherapy

Cryotherapy for the treatment of retinopathy of prematurity is looked for in babies beginning 6 weeks after birth and every 2 weeks following pending getting to threshold ROP or formation of blood vessels of the retina in the periphery. The ones with threshold ROP either got cryotherapy in the places without blood vessel growth in the retina or were not given medical attention. When the person had both eyes affected, one eye got medical attention and the other did not. All of the babies were under 1250g when born. They found that the farther back the zone of the problem was and the more the person had stage III+ , the more there would be an undesirable result. Eyes that had medical attention did not have as many undesired results. Babies with medical attention had less instances of low-vision or blind results.

Optics, Visual Physiology and Correction of Refractive Errors

Contact Lenses

Contact lenses worn throughout the night gives a greater chance of infection in the cornea. The lens may be approved or unapproved for using in this manner. Make sure the person knows that disposable lenses are not less risky than traditional contacts. Wearing either traditional or disposable lenses for lengthened time periods has been linked to a 5 to 10-fold heightening of the chance of getting an infection. Cleaning and disinfecting the lenses properly before putting them in the eye is vital to lessen the chance of getting an infection. Making saline at home heightens the chances of getting an infection. Someone that has a problem with ulcers is commonly found to have worn lenses overnight and/or put in lenses and neglecting the proper procedures for taking care of the lenses with cleaners and disinfectants. Each person that wears contacts needs vigilant education on how long they should be worn, how to clean and disinfect the lenses, indications that come up which may necessitate seeing the doctor and habitual check-ups.

Focal Points

Primary focal point (f), secondary focal point (f'):

- Primary focal point (f) – the place on the optical axis where one object has to be put in order for the parallel rays to come out from a lens. At this point, the image is at infinity.
- Secondary focal point (f') – the place on the optical axis where the parallel rays coming in can come to focus. It is equivalent to 1/lens power in diopters (D). At this point, the object is at infinity. For an eye that has myopia, the secondary focal point is found in front of the retina in the vitreous. The object has to be brought to the anterior of infinity to let the light rays focus for this retina. If the eye has hyperopia, the secondary focal point will be posterior to the retina. The normal eye can focus the light rays from infinity for the retina.

Far Point

Far point in optical terms is the place where the object has to be put on the optical axis in order for the light rays to come into focus for the retina for an eye that is not accommodating. If the eye is myopic, this point is in between the cornea and infinity. If the eye is hyperopic, this point is past infinity or behind the eye. If the eye is normal, it is where the light rays can focus for the retina and the object is on the point of infinity.

A lens to help a refractive problem is decided upon by making the lens one that has a focal point at the same place where the far point for that particular eye can let the light rays at infinity make a focus for the retina. At this point, the image on the far point for the eye is the object.

Near Point, Myopia, Range

<u>Near point</u> – The place where the object is focused for the retina at a time that the eye is in total accommodation. If the object is brought any nearer it will become fuzzy.

<u>Myopia</u> – There are two things that can create this condition. There may be too much refractive strength because the cornea has too steep of a corneal curve or high lens strength. Axial nearsightedness can be caused by a globe that is stretched out. In this case, for every millimeter that the globe is stretched out there is approximately 3 diometers of nearsightedness.

Range of accommodation – Scope of good sight that may be gained using just accommodation. Example: If the person is an emmetrope and has 10D of accommodative amplitude, his range of accommodation will be infinity to 10cm.

When light moves from a lesser refractive index to one that is higher, it bends in the direction of the normal.

Amplitude of Accommodation

Amplitude of accommodation is the whole amount of diopters that the eye is able to accommodate.

If the person is 4-D hyperopic and has amplitude of accommodation at 8, his far point will be 25cm in back of the cornea. He will have to use 4D of accommodation to rise above the hyperopia and make the image come into focus at the point of infinity for the retina. That means there is 4D for accommodation at near point (25cm in front of the cornea). If he is using a 4.00 lens there will be a total amount of accommodation on hand and the near point will be 12.5cm.

If the person is 4-D myopic and has amplitude of accommodation of 8, the far point will be 25cm forward from the eye. He will be able to accommodate 8D past that. His near point will be 12D, located at 8.3cm forward from the cornea.

Different Lens Powers

The distance that the lens is from the eye changes the power. A contact lens is nearer to the eye than a lens in glasses. For example, if a person has a minus lens in his spectacles, moving that lens closer to the eye with a contact lens will make it more minus. That means that someone with nearsightedness will need a weaker minus lens in a contact. Someone that is close to having presbyopia might have to use reading glasses if he is wearing his contacts but have no need for bifocal spectacle lenses. If a plus lens is nearer to the eye, the plus power is lessened. That means that farsightedness will require a stronger lens for a contact than what is needed for glasses. This effectively means that a person in this situation could put off the use of reading glasses for the time being. Also, if a person tends to push his glasses down his nose to read, he is effectively giving himself more plus strength.

Critical Angle and Snell's Law

Critical angle – Incident angle where the angle of refraction is 90° to normal. It only happens at the time when light moves from a medium with more density to one with less density. In a case where the critical angle is surpassed there will be total internal reflection so that the angle of incidence is the same as the angle of reflection.

Snell's law – If light goes from a medium that has a lesser refractive index to one that has a higher refractive index, it will slow and turn in the direction of the normal to the surface. Snell's law will tell you how much the light will turn.

The formula is:

$$n_i \sin_i = n_r \sin r$$

Where:

i = angle of incidence
r = angle of refraction
n_i = lesser refractive index

n_r = higher refractive index

VERGENCE, DIOPTER AND METER

Vergence – The formula is:

$$U + P = V$$

Where:

U = vergence of light coming into the lens
P = lens power
V = vergence of light coming out of the lens

Note: parallel light rays do not have any vergence. Rays that come together are positive. Rays that move apart from each other are negative. Since parallel light rays do neither of these, they will not have vergence at all.

A diopter and a meter are reciprocal measurements. For the image point, measurements are done in diopters. For example, 25cm is equal to 4D and is found with the math problem: 1/0.25 m. Example: object 25cm on the left side of a +5.00 lens, you would find the vergence as follows:

U = -4D
P = +5D
-4 + 5 = 1

So the vergence would be 1D for this object. When changed to cm, this object is 1 meter on the right side of the lens: 1/1D = 1m = 100cm.

REFLECTION, PRISM AND PRENTICE'S RULE

Total internal reflection – When it occurs on the tear-air boundary, it blocks you from being able to see the anterior chamber. To get over this problem, make the critical angle more by using either plastic or glass goniolens on the surface. Total internal reflection is used for fiberoptic tubes and circuitous ophthalmoscopes as well.

Prism power formula: answer is found in prism diopters. Prism power = the amount in centimeters that the light ray is displaced when it goes through the prism. It is measured 100cm from the prism. Light always bends in the direction of the prism's base. Example: 15 prism diopters has displaced light from infinity 15cm towards the base at 100cm.

Prentice's rule is:

$$\text{prism power} = hD$$

Where:

h = measurement of a point on the lens from the optical axis in centimeters
D = lens power in diopters.

As an example, this formula may be used for someone with anisometropia in which there is trouble reading because of hyperdeviation in an eye caused by prism.

Prismatic Problems

Prismatic problems may be lessened with contacts. Contacts, as opposed to glasses, move when the eye moves so that the person will always be using the optical center. This would stop a prismatic effect from occurring. Another option is moving the optical center of the lens down to lessen the h factor in Prentice's rule. A third option is slab off, which is taking some of the prism off in the inferior on a more minus lens. This aids to lessen the prism outcome.

Prentice's rule to find the amount of strabismic deviation for someone with spectacle lenses – for a plus lens, lessen the amount of deviation that is measured. For minus lens, make it more. True deviation will be altered by around 2.5 D% (with D as the power of the lens). For a plus lens, the prism base is peripheral. A minus lens has the prism base in the middle.

Image Jump and Spherical Equivalent

Image jump – Occurs for someone with bifocals; when there is a rapid beginning to prism power located at the top of the bifocal segment. The person looking at something will observe an object to move up at the time that he shifts his eye down to view it. When the optical center of the segment is located on top of the segment image jump will not be a problem. It is more of a problem with glasses that have a round-top bifocal design since those have an optical center farther away from the optical center of the distance lens. Flat-top bifocal designs do not give as much of a problem since they have an optical center that is nearer to the distance optical center.

Spherical equivalent – Find it by taking half the cylinder and adding it together with the sphere. As an example, for –3.00 + 2.00 x 125, the spherical equivalent would be –2.00 sphere.

Image Displacement and Astigmatism

Image displacement – Occurs for someone with bifocals; prism effect that occurs due to bifocal addition and distance lenses used at the reading level. It troubles people more than image jump in most cases. The flat-top lens design is fundamentally a base-up lens. The round-top lens is fundamentally a base-down lens. The nearsighted distance lens uses base-up prism power for the reading level so this person would have worse image dislocation if he has a flat-top design. Prism effects are additive. Also, someone with farsightedness needs a base-down lens for the reading level, so the round-top design gives this person more problems with image dislocation. Someone with hyperopia will have a better time with a round-top design since there will be image jump but the image displacement will be better. Someone with myopia needs a minus lens and will do better with the flat-top design.

With-the-rule astigmatism is handled using plus cylinder at 90°. Against-the-rule astigmatism is handled using plus cylinder at 180°.

Circle of Least Confusion

Circle of least confusion – Someone with astigmatism has two focal lines that are created when the light rays come together (converge). One is closer to the cornea and is made by the corneal meridian. One is farther away and is made by the meridian with not as much power. The circle of least confusion is the circle where the conoid of Sturm is which is (in diopters) the middle of these two lines. The objective for the lens is to get the lens that puts this circle on the retina for the best visual outcome.

To alter plus cylinder refractive power to minus cylinder, add the sphere and cylinder together. Change the sign of cylinder, and then add 90° to the amount of axis.

Thick lenses – Abnormalities that occur include spherical problems, coma-shaped fuzzy places, astigmatism from oblique incidence, chromatic irregularity and warping.

A nearsighted person would angle the lenses to see far away because it adds power. This person should get more refractive power in his lenses.

Astigmatism and Keratometry

Astigmatism following cataract operation – If it is with-the-rule astigmatism, you can look at the sutures that are still there. Snip the 11:00 suture to loosen up the area and lessen the astigmatism. If the person has against-the-rule astigmatism, the sutures will not loosen it up. In that case the only thing you can do is make a loosening cut on the cornea. This person is probably going to be able to use glasses for the problem, particularly when the problem is near the correction that he had before the operation. You can look at preoperative keratometry since this might have been done prior to the operation.

Inaccurate keratometry results – Affects intraocular lens implants in the calculations. Every time there is 0.25D of inaccuracy, there will be an inaccurate calculation of 0.25D. Do the keratometry again whenever there is an average corneal power that is under 40D or over 47D or if the two eyes are different by 1D or more.

Intraocular Lens

Intraocular lens implant – Find the axial distance end to end in millimeters and get keratometry outcome in diopters. Find the wanted refraction for following the operation. Use SRK formula. For a normal eye, SRK formula is:

$$P = A - 2.5\ (\text{axial length})\ - 0.9 * K_{avg}$$

Where:

P = implant power
A = implant constant (according to manufacturer) or may be personalized according to study of prior cases
K_{avg} = average found from keratometry

To find the amount of wanted refraction, add 1.25 to 1.50D. For instance, when an SRK has an outcome of +18.0D (with emmetropia), use a +19.50 lens for -1.00D.

Inaccurate intraocular lens result – For each 0.1mm of axial error, there will be a wrong calculation of 0.25D. Do the A scan again whenever the axial length found is under 22mm or over 25mm or whenever there is greater than 0.3 mm difference from one eye to the other eye.

Magnification Formulas

Red and green light rays with plus lenses – Green rays are shorter than red ones. That means that there is a chromatic difference. This allows for a red/green duochrome assessment. Get the green rays at focus 0.50D nearer to a lens than red. A nearsighted person may be fogged to stop accommodation from occurring, then any red letters will be clearer than green ones. Gradually, in 0.25 steps, add minus pending the green and red letters getting to the same visual clearness. Doing so keeps an overcorrection of nearsightedness from occurring.

Transverse magnification – May also be called linear or lateral magnification. The formula is:

$$I/O = v/u$$

Where:

I = image size, in millimeters
O = object size, in millimeters
v = how far it is from lens to image, in millimeters
u = how far it is from lens to object, in millimeters

Axial magnification – This is the answer to transverse magnification, squared. A magnification on the visual axis results in misrepresentation for three-dimensional images.

Magnification

Angular magnification – Magnifying a simple magnifier, as in looking at an object using your eye or one lens. Magnification = D4. D = lens power that is used.

Axial magnification – Someone with farsightedness has to accommodate more with spectacle lenses than through contact lenses because contact lenses are located closer to the eye and require a different strength. Contacts give this person more axial magnification. On the other hand, someone with myopia has to use less accommodation with spectacle lenses than with contacts. This difference might be noteworthy if the person is in the beginning of presbyopia. The outcome makes the most difference if the person has a big refractive error.

Direct ophthalmoscope – You utilize the eye like a simple magnifier. Round the eye's strength to +60D, then the magnification will be 15 x. That means the retina looks to be magnified 15 times.

Telescopes

Astronomic telescope – Gives an inverted image. This type of image is not very constructive for ophthalmology.

Galilean telescope – Gives an upright image; has many constructive uses for ophthalmology such as glasses lens and contact lens.

Magnification formula for telescope is used for astronomic and Galilean telescopes alike. It is: magnification = D eyepiece/D objective

Note: With noncircuitous ophthalmoscope, a nearsighted eye is like a Galilean telescope. It allows for more magnification. A glasses lens will be minus. The lens on the actual eye is plus. Someone with hyperopia has an eye that works in the opposite way so that there is minification, the glasses lens is plus, and the eye lens is minus.

Four things to help find most useful low sight aid for someone include: most excellent refraction, visual acuity, field of vision, and convenient uses for the person in question.

Bifocals, Loupes, Magnifiers

High add for bifocal – The pro is that it gives a big vision field. The con is that it only allows a short reading distance and that it is expensive.

High-power single vision lens – The pros include that it may be monocular or binocular and gives a big field of vision. The con is that the reading distance is short.

Loupes – Pros include long range for working and freedom for hands. Cons include small range of sight, restricted depth and cost.

Hand-held magnifier – pros include wide range of eye/lens distances and ease in taking it from place to place; well tolerated by people. Cons include small field of vision and problems handling it if the person has spasms or arthritis, but a magnifier on a stand can help someone with these issues.

To find the approximate amount of plus required to read a newspaper with no accommodation, take the reciprocal of the most accurate Snellen finding. This is the same as the amount of plus power needed.

Convex Mirror and Keratometer

Convex mirror – Gives minus vergence, equivalent to a minus lens. By contrast, a concave mirror gives more plus vergence. A mirror that is flat does not add vergence. For a mirror, the power is in diopters, as such:

$$D = 2/r$$

Where:

D = power in diopters
r = radius of the curve

Note: to find the focal length of the mirror, take ½ of the radius.

Keratometer – Measures the middle 3mm of the curve of the cornea. Uses doubled images (done with prisms) to make up for any movement in the eye. This tool will not help to find a scar on the side of the cornea or another fault not in that area. Use a corneal map to find these faults. This tool uses reflecting power for the cornea to find out the measurement of the cornea's curve:

$$D = (n - 1)/r$$

Where:

D = reflecting power of cornea
n = index of refraction for the cornea, which is 1.3375

Geneva Clock and Lensmeter

Binocular high-power single vision lens will need a base in prism. This will supplement the convergence that is inherently already there. If you do not have base in prism the person will end up with exotropia at the reading level.

Geneva lens clock – Tool used to find the amount of curve needed on the back of a glasses lens. It has to be set for the index of refraction of the lens that will be used. A different type is used for crown glass or plastic lenses.

Lensmeter – Tool used to measure how much power is in glasses lens. The lens is put in with the temples facing away from you to get the vertex power in the back for distance. Turn the temples to face you to find the front vertex power (the add). Find any difference between upper and lower segments, particularly when a person is very farsighted.

Retinoscopy, Pachymeter, Hruby Lens, Goldmann Lens, Volk 90D Lens

Retinoscopy – when you get "with" action, the far point will be past the peephole. The objective is to neutralize any light reflex and get the far point on the peephole. Use the light on the pupil to cover the whole space at the same time. Give more plus when it is necessary to move the far point to achieve neutralization. Any "against" action is found when the far point is before the peephole, and the person will need minus to get to the objective of a neutralized place.

Pachymeter – tool to find how thick the cornea is or how deep the anterior chamber is

Hryby lens – results in an upright image; -55D lens

Goldmann lens – upright image; -64D lens

Volk 90D lens – inverted image

Indirect Ophthalmoscope Gives a Bigger Field to Look at Than the Direct Ophthalmoscope

The indirect ophthalmoscope utilized a condensing lens to get the peripheral rays as well. This allows the field to be 25° or more (contingent upon what kind of lens power is utilized). A direct ophthalmoscope has no condensing lens. It can only allow 7°.

Spectrum, Antireflective Coats and Cycloplegic Refraction

Light spectrum – Violet light is at 400 nm (nanometers); red is at 700 nm; less than 400 nm is ultraviolet; more than 700nm is infrared.

Antireflective coat – Put on glasses lenses to interfere with harmful rays; the principle of it is that the crest of a wavelength may be canceled out by another wavelength's trough.

Best pinhole diameter – 1.2mm will counterbalance up to 3D of refractive error; 2mm can only counterbalance 1D; someone with no crystalline lens could have a requirement of =10D and a pinhole to get the most benefit.

Cycloplegic refraction – May be needed if the person is not yet 15 years old, particularly if he has eye misalignment. Be sure to take distances of differences prior to cycloplegia. It may be used for someone less than 35 years old, particularly if there is asthenopia. It also may be used when someone has asthenopia that indicates problems getting to accommodation. Make sure to measure accommodation amplitude and check adds prior to cycloplegia.

Cycloplegic Agents and Vertex Distance

Cycloplegic agents – Atropine will work for one to two weeks (longest). Observe little kids and older people for toxic side effects. Tropicamide (Mydriacyl works for 4-8 hours; it is too weak to work in a child. A diopter or two of hyperopia may be left over. Cylogyl last 8-24 hours, homatropine works for 1-3 days, and scopolamine works for 5-7 days. These are the shortest working cycloplegic agents. Toxic indications include dryness in the mouth, high body temperature, tachycardia, queasiness or disorientation. Handle toxicity with physostigimine.

Vertex distance – Important to find this distance when giving someone glasses that are greater in strength than +/- 5.00D

Glasses for a child who has astigmatism – If sight is not coming along correctly, there may be lazy eye or eye misalignment. Use total correction. Kids can handle total correction more than fully grown people can. Generally lazy eye or eye misalignment happens inside 1.50D of the astigmastigmatism. If it is anisometropia with 1.00D or higher of hyperopia unbalance, it necessitates total correction as well.

Monocular Double Vision

Monocular double vision – May be due to abnormality in the cornea or lenticular area, contact that is off center, improper location of reading add, temporary problems adjusting after an operation for strabismus or lesions on the retina that cause distorted vision (but this is very uncommon).

False positive outcome with potential acuity meter may be due to gap in vision on the macula if the person has lazy eye or a disease in the retina, swelling and fluid in the macula (unless it is ongoing), or an abnormal surface of the cornea (but this can be assisted with a contact lens).

Contact lens – You may need to steepen the fit of the lens if the lens is too taut on the eye. This may be done in one of two ways:

- Give the contact more diameter
- Lessen the radius of the curve

Assessments

The assessments that you should do if someone says his new spectacles do not work as well as his old ones:

- Particular problem, such as far sight, near sight, double vision, uncomfortable fit, etc.
- Measurements from new and old spectacles, using a lensmeter. Check prism from previous glasses. Use cover assessment to assess any unfound strabismus.
- Refraction, which may need cyclopglegic agent in some cases.
- Optical center vs. pupil center
- Reading segments, which need to be even with bottom eyelid. Fit of the new spectacles
- Previous spectacles plus cylinder - assess with Geneva lens clock. Any alteration in base curve; assessed with Geneva lens clock.
- Dryness on the eye
- Vertex distance, particularly with a strong lens
- Pantoscopic tilt, which is generally 10 – 15°.
- Double vision following surgery, particularly in downgaze (caused by anisometropia)
- Strength of the add; use trial lenses to assess
- Size of new lens may be a factor – smaller may be better
- Whether trial frames are comfortable – stroll around and take time so that this process will not have to be repeated.

Hyperopia, Myopia, and Astigmatism

Hyperopia – Acquired hyperopia may be due to retrobulbar tumor, middle serous retinopathy, posterior lens dislocation or flattened cornea caused by wearing contacts.

Myopia – Assess cycloplegic refraction to find out if it really is more myopia. Acquired myopia can be due to diabetes mellitus, sulfonamides, nuclear sclerosis, pilocarpine, keratoconus, scleral buckle and retinal separation, or anterior lens dislocation.

Astigmatism – Acquired astigmatism can be due to a lesion on the lid like hemangiomas, chalazions or ptosis. Pterygium or keratoconus can demonstrate an astigmatism that was not seen before. Cataract problems that are mending can also alter any prior astigmatism.

Astigmatism that has altered – When it is oblique, attempt to turn the axis in the direction of 90 or in the direction of the prior axis. This can lessen the astigmatic power and still let the sphere power stay the same. You can also try a slow alteration of prescription as time goes by to give the person a chance to get used to it.

Jackson Cross, Prince Rule, Hyperopia, and Photons

Jackson cross lens handle – Should be parallel for finding astigmatic axis, but at 45° for telling astigmatic power. The axis should be found prior to power.

Prince rule – Tool to gauge accommodative amplitude

Total hyperopia – Use cycloplegia

Manifest hyperopia – No cycloplegia; a greater amount of plus will make the person's sight fuzzy

Latent hyperopia – Complete minus manifest hyperopia

Facultative hyperopia – Manifest minus total hyperopia; compensation is brought about with accommodation

Photons – Also termed quantums; the extra energy that comes out of an electron. An electron is part of an atom that can get energy from an outside place. An example of an outside source of energy would be heat. Photons have speed of light in a vacuum. When they move, they pulsate and create magnetic and electric results that may be gauged. Photons may also be measured by what happens when they come in contact with the retina. If blue or green is recognized, it is a short wavelength. A long one would be yellow, orange or red.

Snellen's, Electromagnetic Spectrum and Prisms

"E" – At 20/20 on Snellen's eye chart, it represents 5 seconds of arc. This chart gauges least separable acuity.

Electromagnetic spectrum – These are forms of electromagnetic energy: light, x-ray, gamma ray, radio wave. The photons can be measured by wavelength. The outcome of this measurement is the electromagnetic spectrum. Radio and TV have the longest wavelengths. Gamma rays will be the shortest. Light that can be viewed with the eye is around the middle. In the eye, the rods and cones are in the retina. These are photoreceptors. They house pigment that can take in photons that have wavelengths from 400-700nm. Any longer or shorter than that is not taken in and cannot be seen.

Rainbow from a prism – When photons from white light move into a medium that is denser, they slow down and the wavelengths are lessened even though the amount of vibration is static. They bend according to the amount that the speed is decreased. A shorter wavelength bends more than a longer one.

Laser, Nanometer, Rods and Cones

LASER – Light Amplification by Stimulated Emission of Radiation

Nanometer – One billionth of a meter

Rod – Photoreceptor; works at highest quality if the eye is used to the dark; unable to tell colors apart

Cone - Photoreceptor; works at highest quality when there is plenty of light. The three cone pigments include:

- R cones, which are red-catching - 570nm is best (longest), but it also takes in the wavelengths around that
- B cones, which are blue-catching - 440nm is best (shortest), but it also takes in the wavelengths around that
- G cones, which are green catching - 540nm is best (in the middle), but also takes in wavelengths around that

Light to the brain - Photons take in electrical indications by way of photoreceptors, this is given to bipolar cells, this is given to ganglion cells. Horizontal and amacrine cells transform the communication.

Categorizing Color

Color - categorized by:

- Hue - Which means the same thing as color, such as yellow, green, red, etc.
- Saturation - Or chroma, is how rich or pure the color is. If every bit of light viewed by the eye is on the same wavelength, the color is totally saturated. It is a vibrant color. Adding white to a color desaturates it, as in the case with pink.
- Brightness - Or luminance, or value, is how much light comes away from the object to the eye. A filter over an object lessens the brightness.

Primary color - red, green, blue; these are also termed additive primaries since you can make any color by putting the right amount of these colors together (even white). The color wheel is different colors in a circle. The colors next to each other are close in hue. The colors opposite from each other are complementary. Brown is not included on a color wheel since it is actually yellow or orange with not very much vividness.

Eye vs. Ear, Bezold-Brucke and Abney Effect

Eye vs. ear - The eye is not able to find out what colors are put together to make up the actual color that is perceived. The ear can listen to a number of instruments at once and pick out the different sounds. In this way they are very different.

Bezold-Brucke phenomenon - When brightness is made greater, the color will seem to alter. When the intensity is lesser, colors like blue/green, green, or yellow/green will look like they are greener. These same colors look bluer with more intensity. By the same token, red and orange look redder when the intensity is lesser and more yellow when higher. Exceptions are blue around 478nm, green around 503nm and yellow around 578nm since these wavelengths give a color that does not change with light.

Abney effect - When you put more white into a color to desaturate it, the color alters. Every color but yellow at 570nm will look more yellow when you add white.

Luminosity Curves and Lateral Inhibition

Relative luminosity curves - Demonstrate how particular the eye is when viewing various wavelengths of light. It occurs when you get someone to add more brightness of light for different wavelengths pending the time that they look around the same brightness as a yellow light that stays the same. If the person's eye is used to the light, yellow, yellow/green and orange look to be brighter than blue, green and red. The top of the cone's sensitivity is for light at 555nm. This test may be done with an eye that is used to the dark although there will be no ability to see different colors (wavelengths). The rod's highest sensitivity will be 505nm.

Lateral inhibition – If a purple circle is enclosed with a red background, the purple will look to be bluer. If it has a blue background, the purple will look redder. This is because one type of cone gets an hindering communication from the cones next to it.

Afterimage, Black, White, Green and Blue

Afterimage – When you look at one color for 20 seconds, the color seems to get less bright. If you then look at a white piece of paper, the afterimage will be seen there in a complement of the initial hue. This is due to the message that the cones are sending to the brain.

Black – A color that takes in most of the light that comes to it and does not reflect any photons (or very few) back to the eye. This causes there to be no hue.

White – Reflects back every proton in an equivalent way

Green leaves – Chlorophyll in leaves will take in the color blue; red reflects green back to the eye

Blue flowers – Contain pigment that takes in red and yellow very well, takes in green pretty well, then takes in blue the least leaving more blue to be reflected back to the eye.

Combining Blue and Green and Lighting

Blue and green – When you put blue and green light together, it creates white light. That is because they are added together. When you mix blue and green paint together, they actually take away from each other; each pigment takes away a bit of light from the other pigment hue. This causes the paint to become darker than the initial two colors were by themselves, making brown.

> Note: when putting colors of paint together, the outcome cannot be completely foreseen since pigments of paint are not exact.

Fluorescent light vs. incandescent light – An incandescent (Tungsten) light gives out a comparatively higher number of photons in the red wavelength, but a fluorescent light puts out comparatively a higher number of blue and green. This means that colors look different in these two different forms of light.

Blue Sky and Trichromat

Blue sky – Our sun give out every color in the spectrum. The blue of the spectrum is more diffuse than the other colors as the light bends towards people. This makes the sky appear blue. By the same token, the sunset appears red because the earth is moving into more of the atmosphere. This bends more blue and green away and leaves the red and yellow to come through more. This makes the sky and sun look redder.

Trichromat – Someone with regular color sight. 92% of all people can see colors in a regular way. Someone that has congenital dichromatism (a dichromat) has no problem with cones physically, but one of them has a wrong pigment. Someone with tritanopia has a problem with the pigment in the B cone. A deuteranope has a problem with the pigment in the G cone so that it has red rather than green. Deutranopes have problems telling green and red apart. A protanope has an R cone problem that has green rather than red.

Kollner's Rule

Kollner's rule – Very broad guideline; errors done by people that have an optic nerve disease will be more like someone that is a protanope or a deuteranope. With disease in the retina, the problem will be more like someone that has tritanopia.

Hereditary pattern for irregular color sight – If the problem is red/green, it is hereditary in a sex-associated recessive way and is close to being a problem that only males get. Females can carry the heredity and live with regular ability to see, but half of the sons they have will have irregular color vision. Males and females alike may get tritan irregularities since this condition is hereditary in an autosomal dominant way.

Ophthalmic Pathology

Ptosis, Limbus, Trabeculoplasty

Ptosis – Make a cut in crease of the lid. Separate the septum of the orbit and undo it horizontally. See the orbital fat. It is right in back of the septum and right on the muscle part of the levator. As the person ages, there will be another, disconnected medial fat pad that commonly comes through the septum.

Surgical limbus – There is the frontal zone in a shade of blue going from where Bowman's layer ends all the way to Schwalbe's line. Schwalbe's line is the place where Descemet's membrane ends. The back zone in a shade of white goes on top of the trabecular meshwork and goes from Schwalbe's line to scleral spur.

Argon laser trabeculoplasty – See the ciliary body as an observable curved-in area in front of the iris root. Scleral spur will look like a white line in front of the ciliary body. Higher than that will be the trabecular meshwork and canal of Schlemm. The procedure is done on the frontal trabecular meshwork.

Choroidal Effusions, Photocoagulation, Fiber Layer of Henle

Choroidal effusions following a filtering process – Uveal tract is connected with the sclera on the scleral spur, optic nerve and in the vortex veins where the exit areas are located. Fluid divides choroids from the sclera underneath. It keeps the existing associations.

Pigmentation with photocoagulation – You will not need as much laser strength if the pigment in the fundi is dark. The amount of pigment is fundamentally decided by how many melanosomes there are in the choroid. A darker macula means there are taller pigment epithelial cells. They would have a greater number of and bigger melanosomes in the periphery.

Fiber layer of Henle – Located in the outside plexiform layer of the macula; contains associations from photoreceptor synaptic bodies and horizontal and bipolar cells; gets denser and more slanted the farther from the fovea. On the fovea, it goes nearly parallel to face of retina. It is responsible for radial or star-designs of exudate in extracelluar areas beneath pathologic problems that create issues with blood vessels (like high blood pressure).

Blood-Retinal Barrier, Vasculature, Optic Chiasm

Blood retinal barrier – The inside barrier contains the retinal vascular endothelium. This is not fenestrated and houses constricted junctions. The outside is the retinal pigment epithelium. Bruch's membrane is porous enough for little molecules to enter.

Fetal hyaloid vasculature – Three leftover issues include Mittendorf dot, Bergmeister's papilla, vascular loops (95% in arteries).

Crossed/uncrossed fibers in optic chiasm – The inferonasal extramacular fibers will cross in the frontal chiasm and swell going into the optic nerve on the other side. Superonasal extramacular fibers cross right on the other side of the optic tract. Fibers from the macula may be found on the middle of the optic nerve. Temporal macular fibers go through the chiasm and do not cross. Nasal macular fibers do cross in back. If the patient has albinism, a number of these temporal fibers will cross.

Tear Deficiency, Fluorescein Agniography

There may be no tear deficiency following this operation because of the basal tears creation happens due to the accessory lacrimal glands of Krause and Wolfring. Glands of Krause will be found on the superior fornix. Glands of Wolfring are found higher than the superior tarsal border. Cytologically, they are exactly the same as the primary lacrimal gland.

Fluorescein agniography – would demonstrate choroids perfusion and evidence of cilioretinal arteries before showing a demonstration of the circulation of the retina because of the way the dye goes into the area. It goes into the choroids by way of the short posterior ciliary arteries. These are parts of the ophthalmic artery. The middle artery of the retina is another branch of the ophthalmic artery, but it has a round-about path that the dye has to go through. For this reason it shows up later. This time lapse is only about 1 to 2 seconds.

Visual Acuity, Opacity, Ner Supply

<u>Visual acuity for an infant</u> – Since the macula is not totally finished until the baby has reached age 4-6 months, the visual acuity of the baby is not the same as that of a fully-grown person. The region comes to the level of a fully grown person by the time the baby is 6 months old. For this reason, a young baby will not be able to fixate. The ability to do so is equal to the time it takes fore the macula to fully form.

<u>Opacity in the cornea of a baby</u> – Generally is caused by sclerocornea, injury, ulcer, metabolic problem, Peter's anomaly, endothelial dystrophy or dermoid.

<u>Nerve supply source of the lens</u> – This is a trick question since the lens does not have any nerve supply or blood vessels. It is supplied in total from the aqueous and vitreous.

Nerve Supply, Orbital Rim, Cranial Nerve, Anulus of Zinn

<u>Nerve supply of the cornea</u> – The long posterior ciliary nerves come out from the trigeminal nerve and go into the cornea. On the side, 70-80 branches come into the cornea in the conjunctiva, episclera and sclera. The myelin sheath comes off about 1-2mm from the limbus. The network that is in the back of Bowman's layer propels the branch to the epithelium.

<u>Orbital rim</u> frail areas include frontozygomatic suture, zygomaticomaxillary suture, frontomaxillary suture. The orbital bone that has the least strength is the lamina papyracea part of the ethmoid bone.

<u>Cranial nerve V, parts that go through the cavernous sinus</u> – Ophthalmic part is VI, maxillary part is V2.

<u>Anulus of Zinn</u> – A circular area that includes superior rectus muscle, inferior rectus muscle, lateral rectus muscle and medial rectus muscle.

Nerves that go through the superior orbital fissue but do not go through the analus of Zinn include frontal nerve, lacrimal nerve and trochlear nerve.

Innervation, Blepharotomy, Tarsus Thickness, Lid Retractors

<u>Innervation of top and bottom lids</u> – The top lid is innervated from VI, the ophthalmic nerve. The bottom lid is innervated from V2, the maxillary nerve.

<u>Transverse blepharotomy 3mm higher than the top lid margin</u> – You would need to go through the skin, pretarsal orbicularis muscle, tarsus and palpebral conjunctiva.

Total thickness bottom lid laceration 2mm under the lower tarsus – You would need to go through the skin, preseptal orbicularis oculi muscle, conjoint tendon and palpebral conjunctiva.

> Note: the orbicularis oculi muscle was split into three sections by Lester Jones. These sections include: orbital, preseptal and pretarsal.

Total-thickness bottom lid laceration 6mm underneath the lower tarsus – You would need to go through the skin, preseptal orbicularis oculi muscle, orbital septum, fat, bottom lid retractors and conjunctiva.

Lid retractors – Includes capsulopalpebral fascia (equivalent to the levator complex of the top lid) and inferior tarsus muscle (equivalent to Müller's muscle of the top lid).

Lacrimal pump - Uses the preseptal and pretarsal parts of the orbicularis muscle.

ERG – Electroretinogram; used to get an account of electrical discharge that come out of the retina. It is shown with a burst of light. The burst happens when there is transretinal action from ions that are provoked by the light.

Use ophthalmic ultrasonography for the following:

- Assessing anterior/posterior segment for an eye that has opaque media in it
- Checking measurements of tumors in the eyes; checking tumor tissue for marks like calcium with retinoblastoma or choroidal osteoma
- Assessment of a problem in the orbit
- Looking for and finding where foreign bodies are inside the eye

Gauging lengths inside the eye or orbit (called biometry)

ERGs

Electroretinogram; the light is put into the whole retina in an even way in the process called Ganzfeld or full-field stimulation. It generally happens using a bowl perimeter. This provokes an electric discharge from the light. It is made into an account straight from an eye using the corneal contact lens electrode. The sign becomes augmented and is shown with an oscilloscope or may be in writing on the x-y plotter. There has been world-wide standardization for the use of a full-field ERG so that different places may use the same results for research.

The three main parts of the ERG are:

- The a wave – the original negative wave
- The b wave – the positive wave that comes after the a wave
- Oscillatory potentials – little wavelets that could be shown on top of b waves due to the amount of cells located in the midretina's layers.

Other waveforms that could be accounted on an ERG are:

- The c wave
- Early receptor potential

ERGs measure two main things: amplitude (in microvolts, or μV) and implicit time (in milliseconds, or ms). Amplitude of an a wave is found by taking the distance from the baseline to the trough of this wave. Amplitude of a b wave is found by getting the distance of the trough from the a wave to the peak of b. Implicit time is found by taking the time that the stimulus begins to the climax of the reaction.

If there is a problem in retina, ERG amplitude will give accumulated reaction that shows action in the whole retina. This amplitude will be relative to the region of working retina that is provoked. It is irregular if there are big regions in the retina that are not working properly.

Regular, total-field ERG:

- Rod reaction (eye used to the dark)
- Most, put together reaction from rod and cone (used to the dark)
- Oscillatory potentials
- Sole flash cone reaction (used to the light)
- 30 hertz flicker cone reaction

Alternatives to standard ERG include: focal electroretinogram (FERG), pattern electroretinogram (PERG), and multifocal ERG.

EOGs

EOG – electro-oculogram is a circuitous way to gauge standing potential of eyes. It is only available due to the dissimilarity of voltage from the inner and outer retina. To get the measurement, put electodes close to the medial and lateral canthi for the eyes, then let the person move his eyes to and fro in a particular distance. The amplitude will be different for eyes that are used to the dark and eyes that are used to the light. When used to the dark, the outcome lessens and gets to the trough in 8-12 minutes. When used to the light, the amplitude is more and gets to the peak in 6-9 minutes. Divide the highest light amplitude by the lowest dark amplitude to get the Arden ratio. Regular eyes will be 1.80 or more. Less than 1.65 is clearly irregular.

In the retina, the electrical reaction occurs in pigment epithelium. The light peak is created with depolarization from the basal part. To get the EOG potential outcome, you have to use unharmed photoreceptors that are actually touches the pigment epithelium. In the same way that the full-field ERG does, this tool mirrors back the action in the whole retina.

Use of the EOG will be contingent upon how many useful photoreceptors there are. Sometimes the EOG and ERG will both be irregular for the same problem, but that is not always the case. For instance, in the case of problems like congenital stationary night blindness or X-associated retinoschisis, there can be an EOG that is fine but an irregular ERG. Another example: in dominantly inherited Best's disease, the EOG is irregular (with Arden ratio under 1.35), but ERG is regular. The EOG test has a light rise that is just about totally reliant upon the rods. If the problem is in the cones, an EOG will be normal.

Standard Ophthalmic Ultrasonography

An ultrasound is actually an acoustic wave. It is made up of fluctuating particles inside certain mediums. These are measured in kHz or MHz. An ultrasound wave will be more than 20 kHz in frequency. For a standard ophthalmic ultrasound, the scope is around 8-10 MHz. It is so high that it gives out short wavelengths and lets accurate resolution occur for little eye structures. It is different from an ultrasound of the abdominal area that is around 1 – 5 MHz and uses longer wavelengths for going farther down into tissues. This gives a lessened resolution, but it is not as vital since the abs are bigger than the structures in the eye. An ultrasound uses physical foundations of tissue/acoustic impedance mismatch and pulse-echo technology. In a clinical ophthalmic ultrasound, the echoes are taken in, intensified, electronically transferred, then shown so that one can view it on either an A-scan or B-scan.

A- and B-Scans, Lesions and Choroidal Excavation

A-scan ultrasonography – also called A-mode; one-dimensional, time-amplitude way of viewing the results. There is a horizontal baseline that shows the measurement and is contingent on how long is needed for the sound beam to get to the particular interface and the echo to come back. The vertical dimension is dependent upon the height of the spike that is shown. This is a sign of how strong the echo is. This tool can be used alone or together with the B-scan.

B-scan ultrasonography – Also called B-mode; two-dimensional, cross-sectional way to look at the eye's globe and orbit. It shows the outcome in a number of shades of gray, each of which is contingent upon how strong the echo is. Very strong is white, such as with tissue in the retina, sclera or calcification. Weak is gray, such as with clotted vitreous cells. This tool gives a better assessment of problems than the A-scan.

A-scan is mostly useful to look at tissue, and it is beneficial for finding measurements of the inside of the eye prior to a cataract operation. B-scan is mostly useful for looking at the structure, or architecture. Using both of them together is useful to look at where they are the same and to identify the results accurately. These assessments are the most beneficial when used together with clinical assessment and radiographic assessment.

<u>Lesions</u> – Elements that may be found with an ultrasound include topography, quantitative elements (reflectivity, structure inside, and sound attenuation), and dynamic elements (aftermovement and vascularity).

<u>Choroidal excavation</u> – With the B-san, this has to do with something dark on the choroids. The choroids is usually very reflective. The dark spot is a tumor. It is seen when the person has melanoma or another irregularity in the choroid.

Ocular Ultrasound

Ocular ultrasound – Use the immersion method to assess the anterior segment. This is done by putting in a little scleral shell in between the lids. The shell is full of methylcellulose solution. Then the probe is put into the solution. The contact process is where the probe is put right on the globe and may be utilized in assessing the posterior segment. In the contact assessment, every quadrant is scanned in a methodical way. The way the probe is placed is meant to stay away from the assessing beam and meant to keep from making echoes in the artifact-provoking lens procedure. Generally the data is gathered with a Polaroid picture of particular pictures which may be picked out while the assessment is being done, but these pictures cannot give you as much data as is found while the assessment is actually happening.

Assessing Visual Field

Visual field assessments: primary forms are:

- Confrontation visual field – Only finds large problems in the periphery; very basic, anecdotal assessment; person has to look for fingers in the 4 quadrants when he is looking straight at the one doing the test; each eye is assessed separately.
- Kinetic perimetry – Provoking thing is picked out and its location is moved within the field of vision; the region where it can be seen is the target's isopter. Example: Goldmann perimeter and tangent screen.

- Static perimetry – Test location is picked out, provoking object brightness or dimensions are altered until it is either big enough or intense enough that the person is able to view it. Examples: Humphry and Octopus machines

Note: Amsler grid is a tool for finding gaps in vision in the middle or near the middle. When at 1/3meter, every square subtends 1° of the field of vision.

Full-Threshold Testing,12e and V4e, Blind Spots, and Fixation Fault

Full-threshold testing – Static field of vision assessment where the precise threshold for the eye is gauged for each point that is assessed.

12e and V4e – Represents the target measurement and brightness by Roman numerals 0–V (for the dimension of the target in mm^2), Arabic numerals 1-4 (for brightness), and small case letter a-e (for minor filter, where a is most dark and everyone is lighter in increments of 0.1 log units).

Physiologic blind spot – May be found on the temporal field of vision. With the fovea on the middle of the field, this gap in sight is 15° towards the temple and right under the horizontal plane. With a Humphrey visual field, this place has a triangle on it. When you are viewing the visual field, you can tell whether it is the right or left eye by looking at where the blind spot is.

Fixation fault – May be bad fixation, a person that reacts too often, or an error in finding the blind spot.

Errors

False-negative errors – Happens when the provoking object that has more intensity than the threshold is used in a place where it is known that there is sensitivity and the person has no reaction. Generally the person is not paying attention and the problem seems to be worse than it really is. It can also happen when a person has an enormously dense fault.

False-positive error – Since many projection perimeters make a lot of noise and give a sound that can be heard when the tool changes to another position, this occurs when the projectors makes a sound like it is changing but it actually is not and the person reacts. This is a person who reacts too often. It makes the field of vision look better than it really is.

False-Field Defects

False-field defect – the one examining does not notice physical elements and identifies them to be real field defects. Caused by:

- Droopy or baggy lids; lessens the top region of the vision field; tape the top lid to handle this problem.
- Angled optic disc might create a regional alteration with the retina's topography and be seen as a field problem because of refraction. If someone has angled discs in both eyes, it may be mistaken for bitemporal loss of field of vision.
- Little pupil, mistaken for lessened field. Enlarge the pupil first, particularly if the person is having miotic treatment.
- A trial lens rim can make a fault in the periphery for the middle of the field of vision. You can become aware of it when the person brings his head away from the tool during the assessment.
- Any opacity in the cornea, lens or vitreous could create a situation where normal test objects cannot be seen. Utilize more intense and bigger things for these cases.

Visual Field Defects and Pathway

Visual field defects may be categorized by place, shape, how deep it goes, how uniform it is, and how it started and is progressing.

Visual pathway – First order neuron – Photoreceptor (rod or cone), which will synapse with second-order neurons. Second-order neurons – bipolar cells that synapse with third-order neurons. Third-order neurons – ganglion cells, from which axons cross the retina as nerve fiber layer and turn into the optic nerve. The way these are all put together creates problems in field of vision such as glaucoma or a lesion on the optic nerve. On chiasm, temporal fibers do not cross; nasal fibers do cross. Optic tract starts in back of the chiasm and joins the lateral geniculate body in back of the thalamus. Fibers that are crossed go to laminae 1, 4 and 6. If not crossed, they stop in 2, 3 and 5. Retinal ganglion cell fibers synapse to cells. These cells join with occipital cortex in area 17 by way of optic radiations located in temporal and parietal lobes.

Field Testing

The future of visual field testing – Significant improvements for the future include:

- Quicker procedure - Lessen the time it takes to do assessment; 5 minutes rather than the 15 minutes that it used to take
- SWAP – Short wavelength automated perimetry – finds lessened field at a sooner time than the use of the customary white-on-white perimetry; utilizes standard static threshold assessment methods, blue assessment object with yellow for the background. This method can find problems up to a few years sooner than standard static assessment can.
- Frequency-doubling perimetry – Still being created; might be a very important tool in years to come

Eye Drops

Use punctual occlusion, which will lessen how much drains out in the lacrimal system (65% better) which would let a larger amount of medicine stay in the eye. Using the drops more often could also help. A different medicine, bigger concentration, more lipid solubility, or the addition of a surfactant can help. You may also try an alternate way of putting it into the eye.

When using Eye drops from a 50 μL drop, just 20% actually stays in the conjunctiva. The extra comes out of the eye right away (over the lids). From that part that stays in, 80% goes into the lacrimal system. Since there is a 15% per minute tear return, just about every bit is gone within 5 minutes. If the drop aggravates the eye, there will be more tears and the drops will clear out even faster. In this 5 minutes there are several things blocking its pathway. These include the episclera, sclera, and constricted seams to the retinal pigment epithelium. In the cornea, the blocks include the epithelium, endothelium and cellular membranes. These restrict how much medicine can get in. In the stroma, the diluted surroundings restricts the medicine. This means that only a tiny bit can get into the posterior segment when the medicine is given topically. If the eye has flare-up or infection, the obstacles are not as strong and get into the eye slightly better.

METHODS OF DELIVERY

Topical medicine:

- Drops – pro: ease of use; con: length of time that medicine stays in the eye (5 minutes) and the need to use it often; temporary overuse or toxic effects may occur.
- Suspension – pro: longer time; cons include aggravation and tearing as a provoked reflex. The medicine will sit on the bottle's lower section so it should be shaken. People sometimes say that there is a gathering of precipitates in the bottle. Some people do not shake.
- Ointment – pro: even more time for the medicine to work, less need to use it as often; cons include a film covering the eye that makes sight fuzzy. A water-soluble medicine will not dissolve in an ointment and therefore forms a crystal. These crystals get stuck in the ointment pending coming to touch the eye and the ointment melting due to the warm body. It creates a steady flow of the medicine, but the medicine concentration is low.
- Also included: soft contacts, soluble ocular inserts, implantable tools.

STEROIDS

Topical steroids – The particular way that steroids work is only partly comprehended. On the molecular side of it, inhibition of arachidonic acid comes out from phospholipics could create the critical outcome. Arachidonic acid gets changed to protaglandins and the compounds that have to do with it become strong mediators for flare-up. On the cellular side, the medicine has to be taken to the cytoplasm in order to bind to soluble receptors. Then they go into the nucleus and change the different proteins that work for immunity and flare-up. On the tissue side, they push down any indications of flare up like swelling, high temperature, hurting, or redness. It creates restricted blood vessels, lessens vessel permeability for flare-d cells. The cellular and intracellular membranes become normal and stop flare-up provokers like histamine. Neutrophilic leucocytosis is stopped. Macrophage enrollment and relocation is lessened.

These situations (generally) need topical steroids:

- Following surgery
- Immune hyperreactivity
- Immune issue and infection working together

Guidelines for choosing a strong steroid with a quick tapering off time -- When choosing a strong steroid with a quick tapering off time (so that the total time to take the medicine is shorter), remember that the anti-inflammatory outcomes from topical steroids are different and contingent upon the way the medicine is measured in the particular setting. Even so, these general guidelines may be used:

- Bigger concentration, using it more often (even every 5 minutes) – this will give more steroid into the cornea and aqueous
- If the corneal epithelium is fine: prednisolone acetate suspension is better than dexamethasone alcohol solution is better than prednisolone sodium phosphate solution is better than dexamethasone phosphate ointment.
- If the corneal epithelial is faulty: prednisolone sodium phosphate solution is better than dexamethasone phosphate solution is better than prednisolone acetate suspension.

Topical Antibiotics

Generic:

- Aminoglycosides Gentamicin
- Bacitracin
- Chloramphenicol
- Erythromycin
- Ciprofloxacin
- Ofoxacin
- Norfloxacin
- Bacitracin, neomycin, polymyxin B
- Sulfisoxazole
- Sulfacetamide
- Tetracycline
- Trimethoprim and polymyxin B
- Polymyxin B

Refractive Surgery and Sutures

Refractive surgery – Some people need it due to insufficient lens correction, some for personal reasons to eliminate corrective lenses and give the best sight possible. The minimum age is 18-21, and the eye has to be stable. Counter-indications: an unstable eye, bodily issue or drugs that can make it hard to mend afterwards. Make sure the person's reason for the surgery and anticipation of what it will be like are reasonable. For nearsightedness, choices are radial keratomy (RK), photorefractive keratectomy (PRK), laser in-situ keratomileusis (LASIK), intracorneal ring segments (Intacs), or phakic intraocular lens implant. Each of these has advantages and disadvantages, and complications may arise.

Suture methods – Advisable – an ongoing, 8-0 vicryl suture, shutting Tenon's capsule and conjunctiva independently. Use the locking method for Tenon's. Use nonlocking for conjunctiva. Other methods are the 9-0 vicryle suture, 10-0 nylon suture, and 9-0 polydioxanone suture (PDS), which may be in one or two layers. Be detailed with sutures to make them water-tight.

Glaucoma Surgery

Glaucoma surgery – used to lessen the IOP. This occurs when the optic nerve and visual field becomes secure. The objective is to get the pressure to be 30% less than it was before the surgery. Complications include very uncommon chance of losing sight or an eye because of bleeding or infection. Other risks include lessened sight, infection, bleeding, inability to manage IOP, another operation becoming necessary, drooping eyelid, or fuzzy sight lasting 2 a minimum of 2 weeks. As time goes by, complications include endophthalmitis, worsened glaucoma and worsened cataract. A good candidate will have an eye that is usually fine, good outcome in the other eye, white skin color, a phase of the condition that is beginning or medium, and a lack of prior steroid response or previous eye operation. A poor candidate would have prior problems with surgery, non-white skin color, prior keloid formation, blood vessel alterations, misplaced lens with vitreous, irregular sclera, no ability to take corticosteroids, irregular conjunctiva or a surgeon with a lack of experience.

Trabeculectomy Surgery

Fornix and limbal conjectival methods – Outcomes are comparable, but limbus approach is favored if antimetabolites are utilized since it has less of a chance of seeping from the wound. If the fornix-based flab is shut well on the limbus, very good filtration can be the outcome. Many times a scarred conjunctiva means that the fornix approach flap should be done. This has to be done well enough to the back to make sure it is shut a minimum of 10mm (can be more) away from the limbus. Doing so lessens the chance of seeping and scars since the harm done to the conjunctiva can mend away from the flap.

Drugs to cease – Aspirin should not be taken for 2 or more weeks before surgery. Coumadin needs to stop one to four days before when it can be, with the consent of the internist. Carbonic anhydrase inhibitors taken by mouth, pilocarpine, carbachol, and echothiophate need to be discontinued the night prior to the operation.

The alternatives for anesthesia during a trabeculectomy:

- Advisable: facial nerve block with 7ml of mepivacaine and a little, 25-gauge needle utilizing the Nadbath method. Use peribulbar block with 25-gauge, tapered 1 ½ inch needle and 50/50 mepivacaine/bupivacaine including hyaluronidase.
- Blitz anesthesia – begin with xylocaine 1% jelly in preop. Do not use facial nerve block. Next, in the operating room, use paracentesis done with 30° sharp blade on the temporal side, which lets a bit of aqueous out. Use injection of 0.1ml of 1% nonpreservevd lidocaine. Create fornix-based flap using Wescott scissors and smooth forceps. Put an extra 0.5ml in, injected from each direction beneath Tenon's layer. Then go on with the surgery. If the flab is limbal, use a 30-gauge needle instead of 1% nonpreserved lidocaine. Get the person to look down, then put in 0.5ml, 10mm back in a back and forth way. This will blow up the Tenon's capsule and conjunctiva area. When it is being shut, whether fornix or limbus, put an extra 1% nonpreserved lidocaine on cut places.

The Shape and Thickness of the Flap and Size of Internal Block for Trabeculectomy:

Flap – May be a triangle or rectangle shape, contingent upon the surgeon. The result will be the same. Thickness matters, however, since the 1/3 to ½ thicken flap gives better results for filtration over time. Use adequate sutures to keep too much filtration from occurring.

Internal block – When taking out the sample, the generally advised size is ½ - 2/3 of the scleral flap. If a normal flap is around 4 x 2 mm, then a 2-3 x 1mm block is generally adequate. A bigger amount of filtration is had if an edge in the internal block corresponds with a border on the flap. Shut is well and let it go with laser suture break down after the operation. Take out the internal block utilizing Vanass scissors and 0.12 forceps. A Gass punch could also be used.

Paracentesis and iridectomy with filtration operation -- Both must be done during the operation (every time) so that a papillary obstruction will not arise and to make sure the iris will not have a chance to block the ostium in a case where the chamber becomes less deep than it should be. Do the iridectomy as basal and make sure it is big enough so the iris cannot block the place where the trabeculectomy is opened. Take out the extra fluid using a sharp blade on the temporal side or TB syringe and 27-gauge needle. This will be needed to make sure the anterior chamber mends after the operation. Also, the process of filling up the AC gives the surgeon the change to see the flow beneath the flap.

How taut the scleral flap should be -- The tautness sutures are contingent upon how deep the anterior chamber is and amount of seepage wanted. When the IOP is very high, the sutures will need to be more taut and more in number to make sure the IOP does not go too low too fast after the procedure. Sutures can be lysed using the argon laser in 1 day to 3 weeks (or more) following when antimetabolites are utilized. Tauter sutures are needed when AC is not deep. You can utilize more releasable sutures into the transparent cornea since they are simple to take out with a slit lamp. If you are using permanent sutures, the flap may be shut in a medium taut way, then use releasable sutures to lessen the flow even more, and these can be easily taken out as well. If there is a need for more filtration, use argon suture break down. If it is low-tension glaucoma, sutures that are not as taut are fine.

Location of the Limbal-Based Conjunctival Flap and Scleral Flap in a Trebeculetomy:

Limbal – The flap must be done in the anterior. The conjunctiva and Tenon's capsule have to be cut with Wescott scissors or Weck-cell sponge pending the place were zero fibers cross the corneoscleral sulcus. Take out the fibers with the 67-Beaver blade on the 45° angle away from the cut. Keep going in the anterior pending the place where there is no more cleaning to be done. It is too hard to put in the flap when the area is not really cleaned out.

Sclera – Has to be through episcleral tissue. Take out the tissue from exposed sclera prior to creating the flap so that the tissue will not block the flap and make the operation unsuccessful. You have to be able to see the real limbus and the episcleral tissue should be reflected there prior to creating the flap. Cut the flap. Take out the trabecular meshwork since it is close by.

How Deep to Cut the Scleral Flap, Tenon's Capsule, Atropine, Steroids:

Scleral flap – In the anterior, the depth is about the eye: big and myopic eye will be different from a little hyperopic eye.

Tenon's capsule – Some people take it out, but it can have complications. Taking it out is not recommended.

Atropine – 1% may enlarge the pupil maximally and relocate a lens iris diaphragm to the back. It lessens the chance of flat anterior chamber for the beginning days after surgery. It can be used at 1%, 2-4 times a day after the operation if the surgeon thinks it is needed due to the likelihood of a flat chamber.

Steroids – Use prednisone acetate 1% every other hour for the wakeful hours in the beginning week, then 4 times a day for a month. Then lessen it in a fast week for 2 weeks. Use broad-spectrum antibiotic (topical) for a week (4 times a day), and it is recommend to add an NSAID 4 times a day along with the steroids for a month.

Wound seeping – May need collagen shield or bandage contact lens and patch if the seeping is close to the limbus. If near the flap, try patch or cyanoacrylate glue. Sometimes an operation to close is needed for a bleb. A suture break just needs to be stitched up.

Vitreous in wound during surgery – Shut the wound right away and go to an alternate spot. Limited cellulose sponge and scissors vitrectomy may be needed for operation to go on in some cases. If a great deal of vitreous is there, you likely need to do total anterior surgical removal of the vitreous. Losing vitreous happens more often if the eye has no crystalline lens or has an intraocular implant and there is zonular weakening. The eye is more likely to have problems with ocular syphilis, Marfan's syndrome, pseudoexfoliation, homocystinuria, or a lot of nearsightedness.

PRP and Iris Obstruction

Panretinal photocoagulation (PRP) – will not fix sight in a case of proliferative retinopathy. It will, however, help stop the sightlessness that can occur with this condition. Macular focal laser is the better choice to use first since PRP may cause lessened peripheral vision and inability to see at night. PRP also may cause problems with accommodation, enlargement of papillary area and burns on the macula that occur unintentionally. Up to 1/3 of people who get PRP are not helped with NVD or NVE problems. It is unclear whether supplemental PRP is helpful.

Iris obstruction – you can put miochol by way of paracentesis into the anterior chamber to try to tighten the pupil and move it out of the area. After that, inject a visoelastic agent. Use cannula or 30-gauge needle for taking out the iris on the area. Sometimes an iris will not block an atrium all the way so that filtration can happen around the block.

Antimetabolites for Trabeculectomy

Main advance for antimetabolites from the last 10 years is the 5-fluorouracil (5-FU) and mitomycin C (MMC). These weaken ability to mend and help the creation of well-performing filtering blebs. Today antifibrotic agents give better outcomes, but they are restricted in use because of problems that can occur (like toxicity). There is no standard for length of use or concentration. It may be needed when there is scarring on the superior conjunctiva, a prior instance of ineffective filter, a patient that is not yet 50 years old, intraocular lens implant, no crystalline lens, or optic nerve and field of vision damage that has progressed and wanted pressure following the surgery of lower than 14 mmHg. MMC and 5-FU in the surgery can heighten the success of trabeculectomy surgery to 86%-93%. Problems after surgery include suprachoroidal bleeding, choroidal separation, endophthalmitis that shows up later, flat anterior chamber, or seeping wound. It is wiser to not use antimetabolites for a main operation in a person that has a low number of risk elements. Antimetabolites:

- 5-fluorouracil (5FU) – Influences mainly the S-phase of the cell cycle. In an operation with 50mg/ml, it can be put on Weck-cell sponge on the sclera beneath conjunctiva and Tenon's capsule and remain there for 5 minutes. The sclera will be washed using 30cc balanced salt solution. Extra 5-FU injections of 0.1 ml (5mg) can be utilized after surgery when there is a blister that is thick, red and with blood vessels. Generally it is not necessary after surgery.
- Mitomycin C (MMC) – 100 times more potent; inhibits fibroblastic growth no matter what phase the cell cycle was in. Concentration of 0.2-0.4mg/ml may be used. The best concentration and best time to leave it in use is unknown. Some recommend 0.4mg/cc of it using the Weck-cell sponge of 1mm x 4mm. Put in on the scleral, and drape Tenon's capsule and conjunctiva on top prior to creating any scleral flap. Assess scarring and chances of harm when determining the time, which will be 1.5 to 3.5 minutes.

Ciliary Obstruction and Preexisting Filter

Ciliary obstruction – Ciliary procedures frequently obstruct the area if the eye is little and hyperopic, has ongoing angle closure, and nanophthalmos. Following the time when the trabeculectomy sample is taken out, ciliary procedures can rotate to the filtering area. For up to 90% of instances, shutting the scleral flap, reshaping the anterior chamber, and reinstituting regular anatomy will let the ciliary go back to its regular place. If it is still obstructing the area it may be cauterized and removed. Watch out for the vitreous face since it should not be touched. Doing this does not cause much pain and could give the operation a better result.

Preexisting filter – To make sure there is ongoing use for a preexisting trabeculectomy, the alternatives are temporal clear corneal and limbal temporal phacoemulsification. Put a foldable lens into the eye inside the capsular bag. Do the minimum handling of the area so that the filter will keep working the way it should after the surgery.

Flat Anterior Chamber, Intraocular Pressure

Flat anterior chamber – Similar symptoms may indicate too much filtration as the most frequently seen reason. Other indications may be serous choroidal separation, bleeding choroidal separation, papillary obstruction, or malignant glaucoma.

Intraocular pressure following trabeculectomy – If it is high, utilize digital decompression or selective suture break down to lessen it. Beta blockers and alpha agonists are not recommended since it could lessen the aqueous flow. Aqueous flow is necessary for upholding fistula and flourishing blister. If the intraocular pressure is zero and the anterior chamber is not shallow and is formed well, utilize enlarging drops and a weaker steroid. Assess wound seeping. The person should use a plastic shield when asleep. Many times, self- provoked injury can happen and bring the IOP down significantly. When the chamber is formed, watch carefully to see if the IOP goes up during the next days or weeks.

Surgery Necessity and Process

Cataract operation – this procedure is discretionary and depends upon what the person wants and needs as well as the assessment from the physician regarding how much sight will get better if the operation is done. Cataracts may be handed with refraction or papillary dilation as an alternative. Prior to surgery, check sight with Snellen test, potential acuity assessment, or Glare/contrast sensitivity. These do not give the complete influence of the cataract, but they do aid in assessing the problem.

The process:

- Enlarge the pupil
- Disinfect the eye and lids; use antiseptic (generally iodine-based)
- Anesthetize the eye and lids; put speculum on in order to keep the lids open
- Cut the AC
- Visoelastic in the AC
- Open AC to get to the lens mass utilizing capsulotomy or capsulorhexis
- Take out nucleus with phacoemulsification or by hand
- Take out left over cortex
- Put in the intraocular lens
- Suture (optional if it is self-healing)

Cataract Surgery Anesthesia

Anesthesia options:

- Retrobulbar
- Peribulbar
- Topical

The majority of surgeons use local anesthesia (as opposed to general) if it is a fully grown person. Facial akinesia including a short-working agent like lidocaine and hyaluronidase is commonly chosen so that the person will not squeeze his eyes closed in the operation. Cons of using topical anesthesia include action from the eye in the operation (due to lack of akinesia) and the person has to choose topical anesthesia and be able to heed the surgeon's instructions.

Problems that arise from local pain prevention include retrobulbar bleeding (most frequently seen problem due to retrobulbar injection), ocular perforation in a case where a needle went into the globe (more chance of this if there is a lot of nearsightedness and long axial distance), or optic nerve sheath bleeding due to a needle going into the optic nerve (which may cause central retinal vein and/or artery block). The peribulbar injection done utilizing the shorter needle is often chosen, as is topical anesthesia.

Cataract Removal and Phacoemulsification

Methods of cataract removal:

- Intracapsular surgery – Best method from 1752 to the beginning 1970's; found by Jacques Daviel. Uses cryo probe. This method is not normally used currently unless the eye has a dislocated lens.
- Extracapsular surgery (ECCE) – Most commonly used. The forms include manually taking out or phacoemulsification.
- Lasers are not used for cataract removal, but they may be utilized for opening membranes which may form following the operation.

Phacoemulsification – Called phaco; Dr. Charles Kellman founded it in 1967; type of extracapsular operation in which a 3.0mm cut is made through which the cataract is taken out. Since the cut is smaller, sight mends faster. There is less astigmatism, smaller chance of expulsive bleeding and lessened complications with the wound. Traditional extracapsular operations had a wound of around 10mm (15°). This procedure is done with a machine, so it takes time to learn to use it. It is costly, hard to do if the nucleus is hard, and the pupil must be enlarged well.

Capsulotomy and Couching

Capsulotomy – The two forms include can-opener capsulotomy and continuous-curve capsulorhexis (CCC).

Couching – A very old surgical method of taking out cataract, dating back to 800 B.C. as used by an Indian physician Susruta. It was used up to the 1850s in the U.S. It is an eye needles puncture that moves the whole lens back and down to the posterior chamber. This is still used in third world countries.

Vision may be corrected after cataract removal in one of three ways: glasses, contacts or intraocular lens. Note: The intraocular lens was founded by Ridley and used for the first time in 1949. They are made of PMMA, silicone and acrylic elements. The optical part is termed *optic*; the rest is termed *haptic*. The haptic part is utilized when fixating the intraocular lens. The majority are just for distance, but multifocal ones are obtainable too. The shape is a circle or oval. Some have positioning holes and some do not. The size may be 5-7mm.

IOL and Cataract Wound

IOL position – the majority are located in capsular bag, ciliary sulcus or anterior chamber. Capsular bag is desired since it gives great lens steadiness and is not close to the corneal endothelium.

IOL counter indications – Should not be put into an eye that has severe anterior segment disease or flare-up. They are not widely used for kids, but this is changing and kids are getting them more now.

IOL power – The majority utilize the regression formula of SRK to find the power: P=A-2.5L-0.9K.

Cataract operation wound – Has to be shut depending on how big it is and how it was made. A bigger ECCE cut will need 10-0 nylon sutures (radial, running, or mixture of these). Think about astigmatism since a more constricted suture tie creates more astigmatism. The phaco cuts are little and basically will heal by themselves without astigmatism, but a number of surgeons will still use a minimum of one suture.

Following Cataract Surgery

Cataract operation – Following the procedure, medical attention includes a check in the initial 48 hours (24 hours is best) to look at IOP, the wound, flare-up in anterior chamber and location of intraocular lens. Drugs used after surgery include antibiotic solutions to handle infection and steroids or anti-inflammatory medications that are not steroids.

Retrobulbar bleeding – When blood gathers there is can create a rise in the IOP due to the blood pressing on the globe. If this happens, use stop-and-go pressure in the beginning. Gauge the pressure. When it is really high, do lateral surgical splitting of the canthus. That will commonly lessen the pressure. An operation is normally called off if this condition happens.

Cataract wound – Frequently seen problems include seeping or dehiscence from the wound, wound burn, hypotony or flat anterior chamber.

Iris prolapse – When the wound from a cataract surgery is leaking, the iris can get stuck in it and fall or tilt. This causes more flare-up and gives a higher chance of infection. It has to be fixed with surgery. When you can, reposition the iris in the eye. Otherwise it has to be cut out. Use more sutures on the region after this is done.

Bleeding – Hyphema or blood in the anterior chamber may occur. Expulsive choroidal bleeding can occur, and this is the most problematic. It happens when the choroidal vessels break, generally during the operation. The IOP will get higher very fast. The anterior chamber is lost, there is iris prolapse, and the whole inside of the eye can prolapse in a case that is not identified right away and handled. The chance is 0.2%. Expulsive choroidal bleeding is a greater risk for someone that is elderly, has high blood pressure in the body, arteriosclerosis, glaucoma or long axial length eyes.

Cataract surgery – After the operation, flare-up may be caused due to distress from the operation, left over lens matter or bacteria/fungi.

Corneal edema – Commonly seen next to the wound, generally gets better on its own. Medical attention for high IOP and steroids on the area can be used if there is flare-up. If the problem is ongoing, transplant may be done. This issue may be due to distress from the operation, preexisting abornal development of the endothelium or heightened IOP that creates central corneal swelling and fluid.

Vitreous loss – Could be due to posterior lens capsule breakage or fragile lens zonular element. If it happens, there is more of a chance of retinal separation, cystoid macular swelling and fluid or endophthalmitis. More distress from the operation could also create more corneal trauma and central corneal swelling and fluid as an added problem.

Retinal separation – Happens for 1-2% of people. There is more of a chance of it if the person has a lot of nearsightedness, lattice degeneration, and prior retinal separation on the other eye. When the vitreous is lessened in the operation, there is more of a chance of this condition. Since the use of extracapsular cataract surgery, this problem is not as prevalent.

Secondary membrane – This is also called the after-cataract membrane, and it arises due to the posterior capsule becoming opaque. The lens fibers get stuck to the capsule and the left over fibers go through metaplasia. People with it generally are seen as having a worsening problem with sight or issues with glare. It generally arises a few months following the operation and it is not unusual for the membrane to develop for a year or more before it affects sight. The rate of opacity ranges from 8-50%. This problem is not seen as often with newer implants that contain acrylic and silicone instead of PMMA. Do capsulotomy.

IOLs, Glaucoma and Cataracts

Intraocular lenses (IOLs) – problems include using the incorrect power, decentration or wrong location, and ongoing flare-up.

Glaucoma and cataracts – primary issues include:

- The use of miotics for glaucoma will tighten the pupil. This makes the operation harder and many times necessitates the need for surgical methods of making the pupil bigger.
- IOP can be heightened due to leftover viscoelastic matter and flare-up. The problem with pressure can be worse and last longer if the person has glaucoma. High IOP could make more optic nerve harm and lessen the visual field. This could cause the person to lose middle sight if there is advanced glaucoma. It is possible to do the glaucoma process along with cataract operation.
- If there was prior filtration surgery, the cataract operation might have to be done in an alternate way. Moving the place can keep it from harming the filtration area. Flare-up after the operation could make the filter stop working.

Forced Duction

Forced duction is prior to strabismus operation, put the lid speculum on each eye. This is done with one or two toothed forceps. Grab the conjunctiva on the limbus. The eye should go back-and-forth, then up-and-down. Any resistance seen is then contrasted with regular movement. Also look at one eye as compared to the other. It is done in order to identify constricted muscles on the eye. If the muscle is tight, it needs to be recessed. In order to determine the number of muscles to recess/resect, use the angle of deviation. A small angle eye misalignment is less than 20 diopters and can be fixed with surgery on just one muscle. A large difference could need an operation for 3-4 rectus muscles. Recession is done before resection. Work on oblique muscles prior to rectus muscles since they are harder to find and separate on a muscle hook.

Adjustable Sutures, Transposition Process

Adjustable sutures – Methods of putting in and tying scleral sutures for strabismus operations let the muscle be relocated to the front or back right after the operation happens. This way if the person is found with an over or under-correction right away, it can be changed and the alignment can be made better. It has to be done in the first 24 hours after the operation. The use is determined by the judgment of the surgeon. A number of surgeons will not use them due to the range of outcomes that are found right after an operation that might not show what the permanent outcome will be. These sutures are utilized most frequently for someone that has thyroid disease.

Transposition process – Putting some or all of a tendon from the neighboring recti muscles on the place where the palsied or underworking muscle is. It is the best option if there are 1 or more recti muscles that are very restricted in use, such as 3rd, 6th or double elevator palsy.

Slipped Muscle, Adherence Syndrome

Slipped muscle – A muscle housed inside a capsule. When doing strabismus surgery for the rectus muscle, you may accidentally only connect with the capsule. Because of this, the muscle can connect back to the eye and then slip back again inside the capsule. If it happens, the muscle becomes more fragile and there is more divergence. To avoid this, use locking bites.

Adherence syndrome – Orbital fat is disconnected from the globe with Tenon's capsule. In strabismus surgery, there can be a mistaken opening on Tenon's capsule that splits the orbital fat and sclera. Then the fat could get pushed into the opening and stick to the globe. Then the eye is restricted in how it can move. The optimal medical attention is not letting it happen in the first place. Do not make an incision on Tenon's capsule that is over 10mm from the limbus.

Thyroid-Related Ophthalmopathy

Thyroid-related ophthalmopathy (TRO) is an ongoing flare-up on orbit; commonly seen in people who have a thyroid problem in the body. Ongoing flare-up causes scars and malfunction of the orbit. It has occurred in people from ages 8-88, but the average is age 40. It is seen three to six times more often in women. It is not usually seen in children. 80% of people with this condition are hyperthyroid. The cause is not known, but it seems to be associated with immunologically mediated procedures in the muscles outside the eye. A number of theories associate orbit and thyroid with antigens that have a fault with immunities. It is still being studied. Medical attention is unclear since the person could get better, get worse, or remain the same. Radioactive iodine treatments are used except when the person cannot have it. The patient may experience vague indications of sporadic puffy lids and aggravation of the lids along with red eyes. Later there will be a pulled back lid, lid lag, or bulging eye.

How to Overcome Test Anxiety

Just the thought of taking a test is enough to make most people a little nervous. A test is an important event that can have a long-term impact on your future, so it's important to take it seriously and it's natural to feel anxious about performing well. But just because anxiety is normal, that doesn't mean that it's helpful in test taking, or that you should simply accept it as part of your life. Anxiety can have a variety of effects. These effects can be mild, like making you feel slightly nervous, or severe, like blocking your ability to focus or remember even a simple detail.

If you experience test anxiety—whether severe or mild—it's important to know how to beat it. To discover this, first you need to understand what causes test anxiety.

Causes of Test Anxiety

While we often think of anxiety as an uncontrollable emotional state, it can actually be caused by simple, practical things. One of the most common causes of test anxiety is that a person does not feel adequately prepared for their test. This feeling can be the result of many different issues such as poor study habits or lack of organization, but the most common culprit is time management. Starting to study too late, failing to organize your study time to cover all of the material, or being distracted while you study will mean that you're not well prepared for the test. This may lead to cramming the night before, which will cause you to be physically and mentally exhausted for the test. Poor time management also contributes to feelings of stress, fear, and hopelessness as you realize you are not well prepared but don't know what to do about it.

Other times, test anxiety is not related to your preparation for the test but comes from unresolved fear. This may be a past failure on a test, or poor performance on tests in general. It may come from comparing yourself to others who seem to be performing better or from the stress of living up to expectations. Anxiety may be driven by fears of the future—how failure on this test would affect your educational and career goals. These fears are often completely irrational, but they can still negatively impact your test performance.

Elements of Test Anxiety

As mentioned earlier, test anxiety is considered to be an emotional state, but it has physical and mental components as well. Sometimes you may not even realize that you are suffering from test anxiety until you notice the physical symptoms. These can include trembling hands, rapid heartbeat, sweating, nausea, and tense muscles. Extreme anxiety may lead to fainting or vomiting. Obviously, any of these symptoms can have a negative impact on testing. It is important to recognize them as soon as they begin to occur so that you can address the problem before it damages your performance.

The mental components of test anxiety include trouble focusing and inability to remember learned information. During a test, your mind is on high alert, which can help you recall information and stay focused for an extended period of time. However, anxiety interferes with your mind's natural processes, causing you to blank out, even on the questions you know well. The strain of testing during anxiety makes it difficult to stay focused, especially on a test that may take several hours. Extreme anxiety can take a huge mental toll, making it difficult not only to recall test information but even to understand the test questions or pull your thoughts together.

Effects of Test Anxiety

Test anxiety is like a disease—if left untreated, it will get progressively worse. Anxiety leads to poor performance, and this reinforces the feelings of fear and failure, which in turn lead to poor performances on subsequent tests. It can grow from a mild nervousness to a crippling condition. If allowed to progress, test anxiety can have a big impact on your schooling, and consequently on your future.

Test anxiety can spread to other parts of your life. Anxiety on tests can become anxiety in any stressful situation, and blanking on a test can turn into panicking in a job situation. But fortunately, you don't have to let anxiety rule your testing and determine your grades. There are a number of relatively simple steps you can take to move past anxiety and function normally on a test and in the rest of life.

Physical Steps for Beating Test Anxiety

While test anxiety is a serious problem, the good news is that it can be overcome. It doesn't have to control your ability to think and remember information. While it may take time, you can begin taking steps today to beat anxiety.

Just as your first hint that you may be struggling with anxiety comes from the physical symptoms, the first step to treating it is also physical. Rest is crucial for having a clear, strong mind. If you are tired, it is much easier to give in to anxiety. But if you establish good sleep habits, your body and mind will be ready to perform optimally, without the strain of exhaustion. Additionally, sleeping well helps you to retain information better, so you're more likely to recall the answers when you see the test questions.

Getting good sleep means more than going to bed on time. It's important to allow your brain time to relax. Take study breaks from time to time so it doesn't get overworked, and don't study right before bed. Take time to rest your mind before trying to rest your body, or you may find it difficult to fall asleep.

Along with sleep, other aspects of physical health are important in preparing for a test. Good nutrition is vital for good brain function. Sugary foods and drinks may give a burst of energy but this burst is followed by a crash, both physically and emotionally. Instead, fuel your body with protein and vitamin-rich foods.

Also, drink plenty of water. Dehydration can lead to headaches and exhaustion, especially if your brain is already under stress from the rigors of the test. Particularly if your test is a long one, drink water during the breaks. And if possible, take an energy-boosting snack to eat between sections.

Along with sleep and diet, a third important part of physical health is exercise. Maintaining a steady workout schedule is helpful, but even taking 5-minute study breaks to walk can help get your blood pumping faster and clear your head. Exercise also releases endorphins, which contribute to a positive feeling and can help combat test anxiety.

When you nurture your physical health, you are also contributing to your mental health. If your body is healthy, your mind is much more likely to be healthy as well. So take time to rest, nourish your body with healthy food and water, and get moving as much as possible. Taking these physical steps will make you stronger and more able to take the mental steps necessary to overcome test anxiety.

Mental Steps for Beating Test Anxiety

Working on the mental side of test anxiety can be more challenging, but as with the physical side, there are clear steps you can take to overcome it. As mentioned earlier, test anxiety often stems from lack of preparation, so the obvious solution is to prepare for the test. Effective studying may be the most important weapon you have for beating test anxiety, but you can and should employ several other mental tools to combat fear.

First, boost your confidence by reminding yourself of past success—tests or projects that you aced. If you're putting as much effort into preparing for this test as you did for those, there's no reason you should expect to fail here. Work hard to prepare; then trust your preparation.

Second, surround yourself with encouraging people. It can be helpful to find a study group, but be sure that the people you're around will encourage a positive attitude. If you spend time with others who are anxious or cynical, this will only contribute to your own anxiety. Look for others who are motivated to study hard from a desire to succeed, not from a fear of failure.

Third, reward yourself. A test is physically and mentally tiring, even without anxiety, and it can be helpful to have something to look forward to. Plan an activity following the test, regardless of the outcome, such as going to a movie or getting ice cream.

When you are taking the test, if you find yourself beginning to feel anxious, remind yourself that you know the material. Visualize successfully completing the test. Then take a few deep, relaxing breaths and return to it. Work through the questions carefully but with confidence, knowing that you are capable of succeeding.

Developing a healthy mental approach to test taking will also aid in other areas of life. Test anxiety affects more than just the actual test—it can be damaging to your mental health and even contribute to depression. It's important to beat test anxiety before it becomes a problem for more than testing.

Study Strategy

Being prepared for the test is necessary to combat anxiety, but what does being prepared look like? You may study for hours on end and still not feel prepared. What you need is a strategy for test prep. The next few pages outline our recommended steps to help you plan out and conquer the challenge of preparation.

Step 1: Scope Out the Test

Learn everything you can about the format (multiple choice, essay, etc.) and what will be on the test. Gather any study materials, course outlines, or sample exams that may be available. Not only will this help you to prepare, but knowing what to expect can help to alleviate test anxiety.

Step 2: Map Out the Material

Look through the textbook or study guide and make note of how many chapters or sections it has. Then divide these over the time you have. For example, if a book has 15 chapters and you have five days to study, you need to cover three chapters each day. Even better, if you have the time, leave an extra day at the end for overall review after you have gone through the material in depth.

If time is limited, you may need to prioritize the material. Look through it and make note of which sections you think you already have a good grasp on, and which need review. While you are studying, skim quickly through the familiar sections and take more time on the challenging parts.

Write out your plan so you don't get lost as you go. Having a written plan also helps you feel more in control of the study, so anxiety is less likely to arise from feeling overwhelmed at the amount to cover.

Step 3: Gather Your Tools

Decide what study method works best for you. Do you prefer to highlight in the book as you study and then go back over the highlighted portions? Or do you type out notes of the important information? Or is it helpful to make flashcards that you can carry with you? Assemble the pens, index cards, highlighters, post-it notes, and any other materials you may need so you won't be distracted by getting up to find things while you study.

If you're having a hard time retaining the information or organizing your notes, experiment with different methods. For example, try color-coding by subject with colored pens, highlighters, or post-it notes. If you learn better by hearing, try recording yourself reading your notes so you can listen while in the car, working out, or simply sitting at your desk. Ask a friend to quiz you from your flashcards, or try teaching someone the material to solidify it in your mind.

Step 4: Create Your Environment

It's important to avoid distractions while you study. This includes both the obvious distractions like visitors and the subtle distractions like an uncomfortable chair (or a too-comfortable couch that makes you want to fall asleep). Set up the best study environment possible: good lighting and a comfortable work area. If background music helps you focus, you may want to turn it on, but otherwise keep the room quiet. If you are using a computer to take notes, be sure you don't have any other windows open, especially applications like social media, games, or anything else that could distract you. Silence your phone and turn off notifications. Be sure to keep water close by so you stay hydrated while you study (but avoid unhealthy drinks and snacks).

Also, take into account the best time of day to study. Are you freshest first thing in the morning? Try to set aside some time then to work through the material. Is your mind clearer in the afternoon or evening? Schedule your study session then. Another method is to study at the same time of day that you will take the test, so that your brain gets used to working on the material at that time and will be ready to focus at test time.

Step 5: Study!

Once you have done all the study preparation, it's time to settle into the actual studying. Sit down, take a few moments to settle your mind so you can focus, and begin to follow your study plan. Don't give in to distractions or let yourself procrastinate. This is your time to prepare so you'll be ready to fearlessly approach the test. Make the most of the time and stay focused.

Of course, you don't want to burn out. If you study too long you may find that you're not retaining the information very well. Take regular study breaks. For example, taking five minutes out of every hour to walk briskly, breathing deeply and swinging your arms, can help your mind stay fresh.

As you get to the end of each chapter or section, it's a good idea to do a quick review. Remind yourself of what you learned and work on any difficult parts. When you feel that you've mastered the material, move on to the next part. At the end of your study session, briefly skim through your notes again.

But while review is helpful, cramming last minute is NOT. If at all possible, work ahead so that you won't need to fit all your study into the last day. Cramming overloads your brain with more information than it can process and retain, and your tired mind may struggle to recall even previously learned information when it is overwhelmed with last-minute study. Also, the urgent nature of cramming and the stress placed on your brain contribute to anxiety. You'll be more likely to go to the test feeling unprepared and having trouble thinking clearly.

So don't cram, and don't stay up late before the test, even just to review your notes at a leisurely pace. Your brain needs rest more than it needs to go over the information again. In fact, plan to finish your studies by noon or early afternoon the day before the test. Give your brain the rest of the day to relax or focus on other things, and get a good night's sleep. Then you will be fresh for the test and better able to recall what you've studied.

Step 6: Take a Practice Test

Many courses offer sample tests, either online or in the study materials. This is an excellent resource to check whether you have mastered the material, as well as to prepare for the test format and environment.

Check the test format ahead of time: the number of questions, the type (multiple choice, free response, etc.), and the time limit. Then create a plan for working through them. For example, if you have 30 minutes to take a 60-question test, your limit is 30 seconds per question. Spend less time on the questions you know well so that you can take more time on the difficult ones.

If you have time to take several practice tests, take the first one open book, with no time limit. Work through the questions at your own pace and make sure you fully understand them. Gradually work up to taking a test under test conditions: sit at a desk with all study materials put away and set a timer. Pace yourself to make sure you finish the test with time to spare and go back to check your answers if you have time.

After each test, check your answers. On the questions you missed, be sure you understand why you missed them. Did you misread the question (tests can use tricky wording)? Did you forget the information? Or was it something you hadn't learned? Go back and study any shaky areas that the practice tests reveal.

Taking these tests not only helps with your grade, but also aids in combating test anxiety. If you're already used to the test conditions, you're less likely to worry about it, and working through tests until you're scoring well gives you a confidence boost. Go through the practice tests until you feel comfortable, and then you can go into the test knowing that you're ready for it.

Test Tips

On test day, you should be confident, knowing that you've prepared well and are ready to answer the questions. But aside from preparation, there are several test day strategies you can employ to maximize your performance.

First, as stated before, get a good night's sleep the night before the test (and for several nights before that, if possible). Go into the test with a fresh, alert mind rather than staying up late to study.

Try not to change too much about your normal routine on the day of the test. It's important to eat a nutritious breakfast, but if you normally don't eat breakfast at all, consider eating just a protein bar. If you're a coffee drinker, go ahead and have your normal coffee. Just make sure you time it so that the caffeine doesn't wear off right in the middle of your test. Avoid sugary beverages, and drink enough water to stay hydrated but not so much that you need a restroom break 10 minutes into the test. If your test isn't first thing in the morning, consider going for a walk or doing a light workout before the test to get your blood flowing.

Allow yourself enough time to get ready, and leave for the test with plenty of time to spare so you won't have the anxiety of scrambling to arrive in time. Another reason to be early is to select a good seat. It's helpful to sit away from doors and windows, which can be distracting. Find a good seat, get out your supplies, and settle your mind before the test begins.

When the test begins, start by going over the instructions carefully, even if you already know what to expect. Make sure you avoid any careless mistakes by following the directions.

Then begin working through the questions, pacing yourself as you've practiced. If you're not sure on an answer, don't spend too much time on it, and don't let it shake your confidence. Either skip it and come back later, or eliminate as many wrong answers as possible and guess among the remaining ones. Don't dwell on these questions as you continue—put them out of your mind and focus on what lies ahead.

Be sure to read all of the answer choices, even if you're sure the first one is the right answer. Sometimes you'll find a better one if you keep reading. But don't second-guess yourself if you do immediately know the answer. Your gut instinct is usually right. Don't let test anxiety rob you of the information you know.

If you have time at the end of the test (and if the test format allows), go back and review your answers. Be cautious about changing any, since your first instinct tends to be correct, but make sure you didn't misread any of the questions or accidentally mark the wrong answer choice. Look over any you skipped and make an educated guess.

At the end, leave the test feeling confident. You've done your best, so don't waste time worrying about your performance or wishing you could change anything. Instead, celebrate the successful completion of this test. And finally, use this test to learn how to deal with anxiety even better next time.

Review Video: Test Anxiety
Visit mometrix.com/academy and enter code: 100340

Important Qualification

Not all anxiety is created equal. If your test anxiety is causing major issues in your life beyond the classroom or testing center, or if you are experiencing troubling physical symptoms related to your anxiety, it may be a sign of a serious physiological or psychological condition. If this sounds like your situation, we strongly encourage you to seek professional help.

Online Resources

Due to our efforts to try to keep this book to a manageable length, we've created a link that will give you access to all of your online resources:

mometrix.com/resources719/ophthalmology

It's Your Moment, Let's Celebrate It!

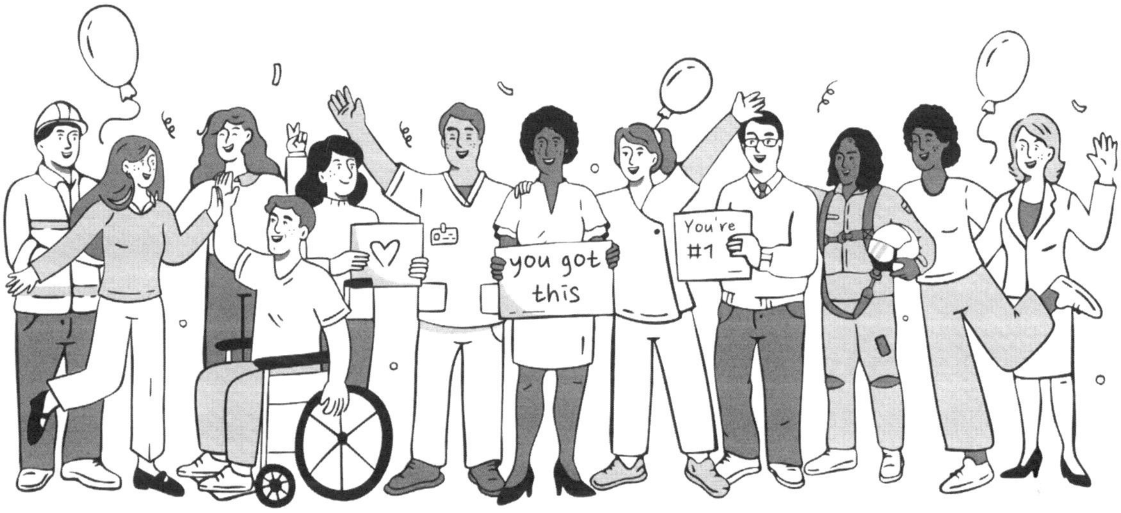

Share your story @mometrixtestpreparation